'Food can play a powerful role in pleasure, health, and celebration ... but it can also be a source of remorse and anxiety. In *Food Freedom Forever*, Melissa Hartwig explores how we can enjoy food yet feel free from cravings and negative feelings. It's a practical, realistic, compassionate – and even funny – guide to establishing a new relationship with food' – Gretchen Rubin, *New York Times* bestselling author of *Better Than Before* and *The Happiness Project*

'*Food Freedom Forever* gives you everything you need for achieving dietary success, for today and for the rest of your healthy life. Melissa Hartwig's information is spot-on in terms of scientific validity, and wonderfully approachable in terms of implementation' – David Perlmutter, MD, *New York Times* #1 bestselling author of *Grain Brain*

'Eating clean can be tough, but Melissa makes it easy! Her philosophy truly works, without counting calories or being a slave to the scale. Her program, the Whole30, helped change my own philosophy on food and how I eat. *Food Freedom Forever* is a must-have for anyone who wants to make changes in their life ... and make them last' – Molly Sims, model, actress and lifestyle blogger

'Step away from the calorie counting, food obsessions, and unnecessary restriction. In *Food Freedom Forever*, Melissa Hartwig delivers a sustainable, healthy diet that will fuel your mind, body, and spirit, and place you in control of your food for life' – Emily Deans, MD Harvard Medical School

'I'm a "real food" registered dietitian who believe the standard low-fat, high-carb, "everything in moderation" advice is complete nonsense. Repairing our relationship with food is critical in order to live a happy life, and Melissa's plan in *Food Freedom Forever* is exactly what does work for my clients. This is no crash diet, and it's way more important than a weight-loss plan – it's the beginning of the rest of your life!' – Diana Rodgers, RD, LDN, NTP

ABOUT THE AUTHOR

Melissa Hartwig is a Certified Sports Nutritionist who specializes in helping people change their relationship with food and create lifelong, healthy habits. She is the co-creator of the Whole30 program and the New York Times bestselling co-author of *It Starts With Food* and *The Whole30*. She lives in Salt Lake City, Utah.

FOOD
FREEDOM
FOREVER

Letting Go of Bad Habits, Guilt,
and Anxiety Around Food

MELISSA HARTWIG

piatkus

PIATKUS

First published in Great Britain in 2016 by Piatkus

A CIP catalogue record for this book is available from the British Library.

ISBN 978-0-349-41484-3

Printed and bound in Great Britain by Clays Ltd, St Ives plc

Papers used by Piatkus are from well-managed forests and other responsible sources.

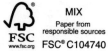

MIX
Paper from
responsible sources
FSC® C104740

Piatkus
An imprint of
Little, Brown Book Group
Carmelite House
50 Victoria Embankment
London EC4Y 0DZ

An Hachette UK Company
www.hachette.co.uk

www.improvementzone.co.uk

For Atticus

CONTENTS

ACKNOWLEDGMENTS

My list is long, but you never know if you'll be in here, so you should definitely read the whole thing.

First, to Justin Schwartz, my editor at Houghton Mifflin Harcourt: Just, like, THANK YOU. After three books and three ridiculous deadlines (who did that?), I only adore you more. Not only are you incredibly talented, but you get so excited when you like something I write, and I'm not sure if you could possibly understand what that meant to me during this process. I'd want no one else in my corner here.

To Bruce Nichols, Ellen Archer, Marina Padakis, Claire Safran, Rebecca Liss, Adriana Rizzo, Brad Thomas Parsons, Jessica Gilo, and the entire Houghton Mifflin Harcourt team, thank you for believing in me, the Whole30, and my dream of food freedom for all. I am so incredibly proud and honored to be an HMH author.

To Andrea Magyar and Trish Bunnett at Penguin Canada, I have loved every single second working with you. Thank you for your enthusiasm, advice, and encouragement, and believing in me enough to take on this project too. Call Mark, because I'd like those donuts now.

To Christy Fletcher, you've been there for me through it all, and there aren't words enough to express how grateful I am. All the late-night calls, reassurances when I needed them most, the tough decisions you helped me make... you're my gladiator in trendy wedge sneakers, and I'd close with "xx" but we're both thinking twice about that.

To Grainne Fox, Melissa Chinchillo, Erin McFadden, Hillary Black, Sylvie Greenberg, and the Fletcher and Company team, thank you for helping me bring this project to life. I am so lucky that people as strong and dedicated as you have my back.

To Leslie Goldman, you are literally the best and I'm so glad I swiped right. (See what I did there? I wanted an exclamation mark BUT I WON'T.) Your insights, humor, suggestions, and red pen were brilliant, invaluable, and probably the only reason I made my deadline. Next time we take a month and work from an oceanside cabana in Mexico; our kids will be fine.

To my family, thank you for believing in me. Thank you for sharing all my media clips with your Facebook friends. Thank you for texting and not calling. Thank you for sending supportive cards, Mom; and grilling the best steak, Doug; and being such a good listener, Susan; and coming up with so many crazy-yet-brilliant Whole30 ideas, Dad; and always being My Person, Kelly (even when I make it hard); and eating English muffins so I can have one when I visit, Ryan. I love you all so much, even if I never listen to your voice mails.

To my #bossbabes: Jane, Jen, Missy, and Tess, your influence, energy, and love make me want to heart emoji. I am stronger, happier, and far more badass with you in my life. To Michael, your good looks were the actual inspiration for this book. I love you almost as much as you love me. For Mel, Diana, Julie, Steph, Stephanie, and Michelle, thank you for being my sanity checks, and for all you have so generously contributed to the Whole30 community. For Ann, I would not have survived without you; thank god you're such a badass because I really needed you. For all my friends who supported me, encouraged me, bribed me, and forced me to change out of yoga tights occasionally throughout the writing process, thank you.

For my BFF Jenn, you will always and forever be the only person I allow to tough-love me that hard. It's for my own good. I love you.

To my talented, passionate, creative, hardworking Whole30 team: Shanna Keller, Kristen Crandall, Jen Kendall, Karyn Scott, Tom Denham, Renee Lee, and my Whole30 forum moderators; you are the heart and soul of our community, and I am so lucky to have you. Thank you for loving this program and these people as much as I do, and for giving so much of yourselves to the community. Take November off.

To Dallas, thank you for creating this with me. The Whole30 community and I will always be grateful for all that you have contributed.

For Maria Barton, I'm not sure you'll ever know how much of you went into this book. Thank you for being so open with me, and inspiring me to give even more of my heart to this project.

Finally, but most important, to my Whole30 community: This book is for you. It's always for you. And what you give me back in the form of your stories, comments, photos, messages, and stopping-me-in-the-middle-of-the-airport enthusiastic hugs is *everything*. I love what we have built together, and I hope this book is all that you wanted, and then 27 percent more.

AUTHOR'S NOTE

I like cupcakes.

Cake is fine. Ice cream is not my thing. Whoopie pies just don't bring it, and cheesecake is damp and squishy and reminds me of the "M" word (*moist*, ew). My favorite go-to yummy treat is, very specifically, a cupcake. It's the frosting-to-cake ratio that seals the deal, and there has to be a generous heap of dense, gritty, so-sweet-it-hurts-my-teeth frosting on top. Like, *inches* of it.

Maybe I should have just said, "I like frosting."

Every year on my birthday, I eat a cupcake (or two). It's been a tradition for as many years as I can remember. This year, on a gorgeous late-winter Saturday, I rode my motorcycle over to my favorite cupcake shop, fully intent on taking something (maybe two things) home with me. I got there, practically skipped inside, gazed at the huge variety of cake and frosting combinations, and ... meh. I stood there debating every sugary-sweet option with the intention of celebrating my favorite day of the year with my favorite decadent food, but when I really thought about it, I just didn't want one.

So I went home.

Turns out, my birthday was just as awesome as usual. I celebrated just as hard. I didn't feel deprived, because it was my decision. I knew that if I wanted a cupcake the day after my birthday, or the day after that, or every day for a week the following month, I would just have one. Because adult, money, motorcycle, and free will.

That is food freedom.

Not the part where I scrounged up every ounce of willpower just to deny myself a cupcake on my birthday. That didn't happen. Not the part where I walked away just to prove how "strong" I was, or because I was terrified of the calories rocketing toward my waistline. None of that happened. Not the part where I raided the pantry later that night because it was my birthday and damn it, I deserved a treat. That didn't happen either.

Food freedom happened when I took the time to ask myself what I really wanted and made a conscious, deliberate decision in the moment. I wasn't swayed by the false promises of sugar, salt, and fat; held hostage by the tradition of birthday cupcakes; or enslaved to a Sugar Dragon who started roaring the minute I told myself I could have a treat on my birthday. I just thought about it, happily made my choice, and got on with my life. The end.

Food freedom is realizing I can have anything I want, any time I want it . . . and in the moment, simply honoring whether or not I *really want it*.

Fast-forward to Easter, a few weeks later. If you follow me on social media, you know I have a passionate love for the processed, food-like products that are chocolate crème eggs. I LOVE them. They're not "special" in the sense that you can pick them up in any old convenience store or pharmacy, but they're special to me. Growing up, my mom would make me and my sister these amazing Easter baskets, overflowing with the usual suspects—marshmallow chicks, ankle socks, jelly beans, dental floss (*See*: jelly beans)—and tucked away at the bottom, one glorious chocolate crème egg. Candy was a big deal in our house, reserved only for very special occasions, so this egg was my most prized possession. I always saved it until everything else was gone, and ate it in the tiniest bites to make it last.

To this day, my mom sends me a pack of three crème eggs before Easter every year. It almost makes me want to heart emoji. Almost.*

This year, on a random Thursday at 2:30 in the afternoon, I decided I wanted one. I unwrapped it, sat down on the couch, sighed contentedly, and savored every tiny bite. I made that egg last a solid 20 minutes, then I texted my mom to say thank you. ("I knew U couldn't wait 4 Easter!" was her response.) It's the least healthy food I'll eat all year, but it was 100% worth it in that moment. And I didn't need it to be Easter Sunday to relive that warm childhood experience.

* I'm also known on social media for not employing tiny little pictures to convey my sentiments. Ever. Thumbs-down emoji, right?

I only ate one, because that's all I wanted. In fact, as of the time of this writing, the others are still sitting on my kitchen counter, not because I'm strengthening my resolve or proving to myself I have willpower. I've just been too lazy to move them to my pantry.

Guys, if I wanted another one, I'd just eat it.

This is also food freedom: The realization that eating something that makes me happy is what *makes* the occasion special, and that "because it's delicious" is a good enough reason to indulge all by itself. I'm the one who gets to decide what's worth it, special, or delicious. I get to make that choice on a moment-to-moment basis. I can think I want one, then decide to pass. I can take one bite, then abandon the rest. I can reach for one, then choose to eat two. I can indulge three days in a row, or not at all for a week.

I get to decide.

You can have this, too, with whatever foods you decide are worth it, special, and taste as good to your mouth as they do to your soul. You can have it without punishing yourself after you eat them, feeling guilt or shame for your indulgence, or spiraling out of control once your brain registers the first hit of sweet, salty, fatty reward. You can feel confident in your decisions, satisfied with your choices, and in control of your own health and happiness. You can free up all that energy you used to spend obsessing over food to focus on more productive things. Like how you'll celebrate your birthday this year: the first year of your food freedom journey.

This is your forever lifestyle.

You can have this. I'll show you how.
Welcome to food freedom.

—MELISSA HARTWIG
March 28, 2016

PREFACE

If you came here from the Whole30 program, you're in the right place. The very phrase "food freedom" was born from your post-Whole30 testimonials, in which you reported feeling happy, confident, and in control of your food for the first time in a long time. You said it felt like freedom; the freedom to eat a cookie and not beat yourself up, to enjoy your vacation or holiday without starving yourself when you got home, to say no to something that used to hold power over you, but no longer does.

I wrote this book for you.

For all the times you expressed frustration in finding balance after your Whole30. For all the times you told me you slipped and couldn't regain your footing. For all the times you asked me for help. This book—a compilation of all the ways I've wanted to support you, my community, in your own personal journey to lifelong food freedom—is for you.

If you have never heard of my Whole30 program, you're also in the right place—but I should explain it really quick, just to catch you up. The Whole30 is a 30-day dietary "reset" designed to change your health, habits, and relationship with food. It's a nutrition program unlike any other; an "anti-diet" that doesn't require calorie restriction; pills, powders, or shakes; or weighing, measuring, or tracking your food. It's been around since 2009 and has proven to be an incredibly effective, life-changing protocol for the millions of people who have completed the program.

But it's not for everyone.

It requires that you eat at least some form of animal protein. The rules are rigid. It demands a good deal of planning and preparation. For

30 days, you eliminate a lot of foods you probably really like—even stuff you've been told is healthy. While our famous Whole30 tough love says, "This is not hard," in lots of ways, it's pretty hard.

But the Whole30 program isn't the price of admission for food freedom.

Anyone can attain this sense of self-confidence, this place of balance, the feeling of being in control of your food for the first time in a long time. And I explain exactly how to do this here, even if you never do the Whole30.* I want you to feel just as welcomed as my Whole30ers, and just as supported in your food freedom journey. I've included an entire chapter dedicated to helping you create your own perfect reset, based on your goals and specific dietary preferences. Use it to change your own health, habits, and relationship with food; then use the tools I'll provide to achieve and sustain your own food freedom.

You've been waiting your whole life for this, whether you realize it or not. And I'm very happy you're here.

---

* Although, spoiler: I'm going to gently encourage you to at least *consider* doing a Whole30. It's just that good.

FOOD
FREEDOM
FOREVER

WELCOME TO FOOD FREEDOM

CHAPTER 1

THE FOOD FREEDOM PLAN

The idea of "food freedom" means different things to different people. Maybe it's eating whatever you want without negative consequences to your health or waistline. (Good luck with that.) Maybe it's giving up your obsession with calorie counting, food restriction, and the scale. (Now we're getting somewhere.) If you ask me, I'd say it means finally feeling in control of food, instead of food controlling you. It means indulging when you decide it's worth it, savoring the experience without guilt or shame, and then returning to your regularly scheduled healthy habits. That's *real* food freedom.

But getting there is hard. Holding on to it is even harder. And creating the kind of balance, sustainability, and control that sticks with you for the rest of your life has always been the diet industry's unicorn—amazing to believe in, but impossible to obtain.

Until now.

I'm going to show you exactly how to discover food freedom for yourself, no matter how out of control you feel right now. I'll point you down a self-directed path that keeps you in control, satisfied, and looking and feeling your best, without requiring that you obsess about food, count calories, or starve yourself. I'll teach you how to cultivate a healthy relationship with food for the rest of your life. And at no point will you have to be a perfect eater, because being held to a standard of perfection goes against the very definition of "food freedom."

The plan is outlined in three simple steps: engaging your reset, finding your balance, and recovering from slips. It's designed to run in a cycle, one step feeding the next, empowering you to create the perfect eating plan for you—one that feels satisfying and sustainable while still delivering the health benefits you want. Here is the plan:

THE FOOD FREEDOM 3-STEP PLAN

STEP 1: Reset your health, habits, and relationship with food.

STEP 2: Enjoy your food freedom.

STEP 3: Acknowledge when you're starting to slip.

Repeat as needed.

Um, yep. That's it. (Told you it was simple.) It's an ever-improving cycle; get in control → strengthen your new healthy habits and find your balance → lose control → get back in control.

Yes, I did say "lose control."

One of the reasons most other diet programs don't actually work in the long term is their promise that once you complete the program—poof!—you'll be changed forever. No more cravings, no more unhealthy habits, no more dieting. Ever.

That is incredibly unrealistic.

No short-term dietary intervention—not even the Whole30—has the power to completely and permanently overwrite decades of less-than-stellar health habits and a dysfunctional relationship with food. And even if it did, when stress enters the picture, those cravings, bad habits, and dependence on comfort foods inevitably return with a vengeance.

So yes, part of the Food Freedom plan includes you falling off the wagon, because you will, and I want to prepare you for that. What you are embarking upon is a constant cycle of progression, but it's not linear. You'll do well, then stumble. You'll be in control, then fall back into old habits. You'll have weeks of effortless balance, followed by (surprise!) a week of Carb-a-Palooza.

This is all totally okay.

Because unlike all those times you dieted and failed, this time it's not failure; it's just part of the process. This time, you'll see slips as a valuable learning experience. This time, you will have a plan to recover. And because of that, you won't beat yourself up about it—you'll simply acknowledge where you are, reactivate your reset, and regain control.

The best part about this plan is that each time you run through the cycle (reset, achieve food freedom, start to slip, reset again), your time spent off the rails will be shorter, and the time you're able to stay in control, enjoying the benefits of food freedom, will extend. Until eventually, ideally, you won't need a reset at all; you'll just be living each day according to your definition of food freedom.

I've been successfully following this food freedom strategy, fueled by periodic Whole30 resets, for more than seven years. If a holiday, vacation, or stressful event throws me off my healthy eating game for too long, I simply acknowledge that my habits have slipped, and come back to the Whole30 as my chosen method of reset. I no longer experience guilt when eating less-healthy food, and I no longer beat myself up for my "transgressions." Even when I do slip or purposefully go off-plan, I never stray too far, my out-of-balance times are short, and the amount of time I need to reset is just a few days. The rest of the year, I'm totally in balance, indulging when it's worth it and savoring every bite, but still feeling confident, healthy, and in control.

Yes, I still eat French fries. And my mom's chocolate chip walnut cake. And yes, even those decidedly un-food-like chocolate crème eggs, because they remind me of home, and eating one makes me really happy. These foods are all part of my own self-created Food Freedom plan, and I've figured out how to work them into my life in a way that feels healthy and satisfying, but still lets me meet every single one of my health and fitness goals. The takeaway:

Food freedom doesn't demand that you always eat perfectly.

In fact, just the opposite. Food freedom understands that you won't eat perfectly all the time; that you'll make poor choices in the excitement of a party, overindulge while on vacation in Italy, and fall off your healthy eating wagon at Thanksgiving. In fact, possibly for the first time in the history of a "diet," those expectations are built right in. Which means you're committing to a plan that actually makes sense, because I'm not afraid to acknowledge what you already know:

You will not always make good choices. Your healthy habits will eventually slip. You will, at some point, once again find yourself not entirely in control of your food. So let's just work *with* that idea instead of *against* it.

Doesn't that feel better?

Your Food Freedom Journey

Here's a more detailed preview of how the Food Freedom plan works:

I'll give you various options for your reset—the short-term eating plan that will catalyze and support new, healthy habits. Your reset will show you exactly how food affects your unique body and mind, change your relationship with food, and allow you to settle into an effortless new normal. For some people, this reset will be the Whole30; for others, it will be a customized program, tailored to your specific goals, health conditions, or dietary needs.

I'll offer strategies for dealing with temptation, creating awareness around your habits, and spotting your specific "I ate the whole bag of chips" triggers before they're pulled. You'll learn a new language around food, banishing guilt and shame from your food vocabulary and taking the morality ("This food is good, but I'm bad when I eat this") out of your choices. I'll also outline the five reasons you're likely to fall off the rails and back into old unhealthy habits, and give you a plan for managing special occasions, social pressures, and stress.

Most important, I'll tell you how to gracefully recover from slips and reactivate your reset, keeping you on track with your health goals and feeling in control.

There's also an entire section devoted to communicating with friends and family about your new, healthy lifestyle, because changing the food you put on your plate often changes your relationships (and not always for the better).

6 FOOD FREEDOM FOREVER

YOUR NEW WAY OF EATING

'll hammer this home again and again: The Food Freedom plan is not a *diet*, it's a *re-education*. You'll be conducting your own research, applying what you've learned, and holding yourself accountable every single day. Unlike other dietary crash courses, you'll actually learn this material, and you (and your body) will retain it for the rest of your life. If food freedom had a Twitter account, its bio would read: "@FoodFreedomForever: Teaching you to be in control of the food you eat. No: Calorie counting; deprivation; ice-cream-as-therapist. Yes: Health, satisfaction, sustainability. And still sometimes ice cream." However, you'll notice that I sometimes refer to the Food Freedom plan as a "diet." When that happens, I'm simply using it as a synonym for "your new way of eating." In fact, once you adopt the food freedom plan, "diet" will take on a whole new meaning—one that doesn't make you anxious, irritable, or hungry.

By the last page of this book, you'll have a detailed map for creating a short-term protocol that's maximally effective, helping you to discover the perfect diet for you, find your own form of balance, and maintain control in a world full of stress and temptation. Sound too good to be true? I promise it's not. But that's where this book differs from all the other diet books you've read. You know, the ones that toss around words like "effortless" and "fast" and swear that all your undesirable stuff (sugar cravings, extra weight, bad habits) will simply "melt away"? They promise that if we only buy the right book/try the right program/find the right expert, we won't have to work that hard at all.

You and I both know that's not true.

Here's a not-so-secret secret: There are no shortcuts. Quick fixes don't exist. There is no 7-Day Get Skinnier Than Your Friends Diet that will magically translate into truly good-for-you habits that last a lifetime. Which brings us to the first piece of tough love you'll encounter in this book.

This will be hard.

While you go through the process, you'll feel like your decisions around food are taking up too much of your time, your energy, your emotional capacity.

They are. It's temporary.

You'll wonder if you're going to have to pay this much attention to what you eat for the rest of your life.

You won't. It gets easier.

You'll fear that you won't be able to retain the amazing results of your reset once you're back in the real world.

You can. You'll find your balance.

You'll be nervous that family and friends won't understand that your relationship with food is truly different now.

They may not. I'll help you here.

So yes, it requires some effort, as all good things do. And it will take time, as all good things do. Which bring us to Tough Love #2:

It's not going to happen overnight.

Or in a month. Or maybe even a year. Discovering food freedom is a lifelong journey of purposeful evaluation, increased self-awareness, and commitment to the process. You can't completely erase decades of bad habits and emotional relationships with food with one 30-day reset. You will spend many months on this path taking three steps forward and two steps back. The important thing is recognizing you're always a step ahead of where you were, and acknowledging that even one step is progress.

THE FOOD FREEDOM CYCLE

Here's a real-life example of the cycle in action: Your goal is to tame your Sugar Dragon (the one who breathes fire in the form of uncontrollable cravings), so you take on the Craving-Buster Reset. You spend 30 days resetting your health, habits, and relationship with food, and end the reintroduction period feeling confident and in control, your Sugar Dragon lulled to sleep in his cave. Then you go on vacation. By the end of your trip, your energy is nonexistent, your belly is puffy, and your Sugar Dragon has awoken with a vengeance. When you get home, you admit that your healthy habits are in serious jeopardy, so you return to your reset until you regain your energy, lose the bloat, and feel back in control. You mentally log what you've learned from the experience ("Wine + sugar = a vicious combination"; "I should still be making conscientious food decisions even if I am on vacation"; "I feel much better without bread in my life, even in the Bahamas") and go on with your food freedom self. I see no failure here, do you?

But as I'll continue to remind you, this plan is different from every diet you've tried. You don't run through this program once and "graduate" with no idea of what happens next. There isn't a "start" and a "stop." This three-step plan runs on an ever-evolving cycle. You'll reset, find your balance, experience what it feels like to go off-balance, and reset again . . . but even though you'll keep returning to the reset whenever you need it, the difference here is that going back to the start is not indicative of failure—it's just *part of the process* (and progress).

Each repeat of this cycle brings you even more awareness, even more ease in making conscious decisions; an even better plan for managing stressful situations and identifying your triggers before they're pulled. You'll spend more time experiencing food freedom, and return to your reset less and less frequently—spending the majority of your days just living, fully in control of the foods you are eating. It's a cycle of continuous improvement that brings you legitimate food freedom every day you follow the plan.

It works if you work it. Here's how I know.

CHAPTER 2

MY STORY

Confession: I have never been overweight.
Now you're rolling your eyes, about to text the friend
who recommended this book, "OMG what could this
lady POSSIBLY know about feeling out of control and
desperate for freedom?" Please don't, not yet. Trust me
when I say I have fought my fair share of battles.

We All Have Our Baggage

Hi. My name is Melissa, and I am a drug addict. (*"Hi, Melissa."*)

You probably weren't expecting that, were you?

I started using drugs my freshman year of college; a year later, I was legitimately addicted. For the next five years, I hung out with a bad crowd and made bad decisions; I lived on coffee, sugar, and desperation. I wasn't sleeping, I wasn't eating, my behavior became increasingly erratic, and it wasn't long before family and friends were officially fed up.

Eventually, so was I. And thanks to the support of people who loved me, counseling, and therapy, I got clean. But I knew that in order to stay that way, I'd need to change every aspect of my day-to-day existence—friends, clothing, music, hangouts, and habits—and most important, change the way I thought about myself.

I adopted a growth mind-set: an optimistic outlook in which I believed that my personal traits were transformable, not fixed. (More on this on page 104.) I mantra'd nonstop that I was a good person, a worthy person, a healthy person. I began running and going to the gym. I changed my diet to include more low-fat health foods, salads, and protein shakes. I made like-minded friends who didn't use drugs or drink excessively. I found a new job, and was quickly promoted to manager of a small department. I tentatively started rebuilding trust with my family.

It wasn't all sunshine, rainbows, and ponies, however. Underneath it all, I still struggled . . . just not with drugs.

I was eating a healthier diet overall, but subconsciously using food to distract, numb, or punish myself. I lived alone: the perfect breeding ground for weighing, measuring, and tracking every bite that went into my mouth, all in the virtuous pursuit of health. I would ruthlessly restrict all sweets when I needed an extra sense of control, yet turn around and secretly reward myself with junk food I told myself I had earned after a few "good" days. I bounced between these two places for years, never quite settling into a healthy balance or questioning my belief that when I ate well, I was "good" and when I didn't, I was "bad." I overtrained, replacing my total commitment to drugs with total commitment to exercise. I got pretty skinny and was tired all the time, totally obsessed with every perceived ounce of fat on my body. But everyone told me I looked amazing and applauded my dedication, so I high-fived myself for turning my life around and swore I'd tighten up my diet even more.

I wasn't using, but this wasn't healthy. I just didn't realize it.

In April 2009, after yet another grueling training session, I was eating lunch with Dallas (who eventually became my Whole30 cofounder). He had been considering the idea of taking on a short-term, squeaky-clean diet as a challenge and asked if I wanted to try it with him for 30 days, just to see what would happen.

I was crushing some Thin Mints at the time, because we had just finished exercising, and I deserved them.

"Yeah, yeah, sure," I mumbled through a mouthful of cookies. "When should we start?"

"How about right now?" he said, part question, part dare. I rolled my eyes, handed the rest of my Thin Mints to a friend, and began. I agreed only to see if changing my diet would help my athletic performance. Never in a million years did I suspect that the experience would completely transform how I felt about food and my body. That self-created 30-day diet experiment turned out to be the very first Whole30.

In those 30 days, I became aware of how often I was using food as punishment or reward. Without access to the carb-dense processed foods I had relied on, I was forced to find other ways to self-soothe, comfort myself, and relieve anxiety. I learned how some of the "healthy" foods I'd been eating were having an adverse impact on my health, mood, and self-confidence. (*Hello*, midmorning snack of low-fat yogurt, eight almonds, and half a whole-grain blueberry muffin.) And I finally acknowledged the subtle ways I had replaced drugs with food, using sugar and treats to numb or distract myself instead of acknowledging and working through my feelings.

The Whole30 changed my life and brought me to a truly healthy relationship with food and my body—a relationship I've been able to maintain ever since. As of today, I've been clean for over 16 years and living in food freedom for more than seven.

Pizza, Heroin, Sugar, Cigarettes

My guess is that if you chose this book for yourself, you fall into one of two relationships with food. The first is a serious love-hate connection: You're stuck in a cycle of overconsumption, momentary relief, self-loathing, and shame, followed by (inexplicably) craving more of the very thing that's destroying your health, relationships, and self-worth. You hide your behaviors, lie to yourself and others about your habits, and believe you are alone in your struggles. You feel powerless over food.

But maybe this isn't your context. Maybe you aren't overly preoccupied with food, and don't consider your pantry a war zone. People in the second category may read this and think, "I'm not that bad. This program isn't for me." I assure you, it is. Here's the thing: You don't have to hit rock bottom to want to improve your health, habits, or relationship with food. Do you have some food habits you'd rather not continue? Do your food choices sometimes slip so far away from you that you feel embarrassed? Do you yo-yo between eating "pretty healthy" and "not so healthy," unable to find a middle ground? (I won't even bother asking you if you're happy with your waistline, because that's not the point.)

Food freedom isn't just for those who need rescuing from the throes of sugar addiction. It's for anyone who wants to create a truly healthy relationship with food, built on habits that last a lifetime. And you certainly don't have to be locked in a bathroom with a box of powdered donuts to want *that*.

And don't forget, I'm right there with you.

I've had Whole30ers comment on advice I've posted on social media, "Please. Look at you. It's easy for you to say, you have no idea what it's like." But I do, because I've been where you are. My history, combined with my personal experience with the Whole30 program, has given me a unique understanding of addictions, fixations, and unhealthy relationships with food; something you can't see when you look at my photo on the back of this book. Of course, drugs and food aren't exactly the same—most people's soda habit wouldn't require a rehabilitation clinic to kick. But the consequences of feeling out of control, whether it's with drugs or food, are actually quite similar.

Like many Whole30 followers, I'd also attempted just about every diet out there before finding a program that actually fit, so we have that in common, too. I tried Atkins, the Zone, one that involved a horrid concoction of "detox" ingredients three times a day, and a few bodybuilding diets that demanded I prioritize shakes and pills over real food. I never needed to lose weight, but once I started exercising, I was forever trying to "lean out," and when you have a dysfunctional relationship with food, eating too much one day often leads to calorie restriction the next. (Paying penance for my dietary sins, as if my food choices were a moral failing. This was what I used to believe.) My relationships with food and my body were unhealthy, counterproductive, and could basically be summed up with the sad face + thumbs-down emojis.

That's how I know that diets don't work—well, that, and the dozens of scientific studies that definitively conclude that dieting (calorie restriction) doesn't succeed in the long term for either weight loss or getting healthier. Every time I tried a new diet, I'd stick to it for a while, then fall off the wagon hard. I'd come out the other side feeling like a failure for my lack of willpower, then go eat some comfort food just to make myself feel better.

It wasn't my fault—and if this sounds like your story, it isn't your fault, either. Dieting is not the answer, yet we continue to fall victim to the cycle, seeking quick fix after quick fix because it is the only thing we know how to do.

Maybe that's the problem.

It's time to develop a healthy relationship with the very thing holding you hostage. It's time to turn cravings, addictions, and yo-yo patterns into a healthy, balanced relationship; staying happy, healthy, and in-control while allowing yourself the pleasure and reward of worth-it foods. It's time to lose the guilt, lose the powerlessness, lose the idea of food (or you) being "good" or "bad" based on what's on your plate or the number that shows up on your scale.

The Food Freedom plan is not based on a diet at all, because diets can't give you freedom.

CHAPTER 3

DIETS DON'T WORK

Here's how every diet you've ever tried has turned out. (You could write this section as well as I did, I'm guessing.) You white-knuckle your way through the diet, forced to expend precious willpower making hard decisions dozens of times a day, because you're not being supported and you weren't given a plan to actually change your habits, your tastes, or the way you think about food. As your willpower dips lower and lower, you have a harder time resisting temptation, and find yourself daydreaming about the day it's over, when you can finally give in and eat all the things you've been missing.

You spend the entirety of the diet paying attention to nothing but the rules, consciously overriding your body's natural signals (Hey, *I'm kind of hungry. Yeah, so, definitely hungry . . . REALLY FREAKIN' HUNGRY OVER HERE.*) to adhere to the plan and ignoring anything that might be suffering as a result. Like your energy, cravings, sleep, mood, relationship with food, or general likeability as rated by your significant other, best friend, and co-workers. You just step on that scale every morning crossing your fingers, your self-confidence hanging in the balance.

And yes, you lose weight—but let's not celebrate just yet. The fact is, your metabolism is actually slower than it used to be, because the stress of the diet changed both your hormones (which regulate your blood sugar, body fat levels, and appetite), and how effectively you burn calories. You're hungrier than you were before the diet, and your cravings are stronger than ever because you've been deprived of energy and forced to overdraw your will-power bank. For weeks now, you've been cranky, less motivated to exercise, and maybe, if truth be told, a little bit depressed . . . but hey, at least you're skinnier! (Oh, but also softer, since crash diets tend to burn muscle mass as well as fat.) And once the diet is over, you're left wondering, "Now what?"

But WAIT.

First, because you succeeded and lost weight, you deserve a treat, and surely you can afford to relax a little because you've been *so good*, right? And since you didn't change your habits or learn how to comfort or treat yourself in a new way, you go right back to rewarding yourself with the unhealthy food your brain has been demanding . . . the same stuff that got you into trouble in the first place. The same stuff that made you gain weight before and will make you gain weight even faster now because your body sucks at burning calories and wants to replenish your fat stores fast, post-"starvation."

And slowly but surely, you slide right back into your old habits and regain all the weight (and then some), feeling like a failure and eating even more to compensate for the stress, guilt, and shame. Essentially, your diet has left you heavier, sadder, and even less healthy than before.

Thanks for nothing, diet. Let's not do that again.

Dieting: Just (Don't) Do It

What do we all want out of a "diet?" Surprisingly, "weight loss" is no longer the most common answer. According to a November 2015 Gallup poll, the number of Americans who want to lose weight is on the decline, despite the increase in obesity rates seen over the last decade. Why the disconnect?

With more than 1 in 3 U.S. adults in the "obese" category, perhaps your extra 20 pounds of fluff seems normal when you look around. Or maybe after doing fad diet upon fad diet without lasting results, you're so demoralized that you've simply accepted where you are, afraid to try something new and fail yet again.

You know what I think?

I think it's because you actually want *more* out of a diet than just weight loss, and the diet industry has its fingers in its ears, saying, "La la la la la." It wants to sell books, powders, pills, and shakes, and the promise of fast and easy weight loss is the flashiest marketing technique. It banks on you feeling bad about yourself, because a lack of confidence ensures repeat customers. It's uninterested in connecting with you as a person, unwilling to guide you through the examination of your emotional relationship with food and how that factors into your health goals. It takes for granted (because it's convenient) that the only thing you care about is your body composition—that improving your energy, sleep quality, chronic pain, medical condition, and quality of life aren't as important as how much you weigh.

That's rude, and it's assumptive. The diet industry is not giving you anywhere near enough credit.

You don't want quick fixes that won't last. You don't want to lose the same 10 pounds over and over again. You don't want to be a slave to the scale, allowing it to dictate your self-esteem or self-worth. And you're tired of feeling like a failure when yet another diet doesn't stick (leading you to eat even more junk food to make yourself feel better).

You want more.

You want to use a new diet as a springboard; a jump-start to healthy habits that will last a lifetime. You want more energy, more restful sleep, fewer cravings, better digestion, resolution of aches and pains, and happier checkups with your doctor. Would you be psyched if you also dropped a pant size or two? Absolutely. But *that's not all you want.*

Ultimately, you want to end the program feeling in control of your food, able to use the tools you've learned to maintain that control long after the "diet" part is technically over. If you could only achieve that one thing— lasting food freedom—wouldn't your other goals (improved health, better self-confidence, and yes, a trimmer waistline) be that much easier to achieve?

Unfortunately, every diet you've tried in the past has failed to bring you long-term results because they do everything you *don't* want them to do, and very little of what you actually *need*. First, they offer only a temporary quick fix, promising you'll lose weight fast without any plan to help you keep it off. As a result, the scale is your only metric for success, which discourages you from focusing on the other potentially life-changing benefits of improving your diet and making yourself healthier.

In addition, diets almost always depend on calorie restriction, which often requires counting, measuring, or tracking your food: a tedious, unsustainable practice. And because they often don't delve into the *why* of the program, connecting with you intellectually and emotionally and providing you with internal motivation to stick with it, you're forced to rely on sheer willpower to survive the program.

WILLPOWER

Did you know that willpower is a finite resource? This means that, despite your diet's encouragement to "buckle down" and "stay strong," you will, at some point, run out. Lots of things tap our willpower bank, like biting your tongue when your boss says something stupid, ignoring the ping of a new e-mail, or resisting the candy on your co-worker's desk. Willpower is highest in the morning, but quickly runs low throughout the day when you're dieting, as you're forced to resist the signals your body is sending you in favor of sticking to the plan. Is it any wonder that we tend to impulse shop, gamble, or binge-watch Netflix more when we're on a diet? This may explain why, once the diet is over, you simply can't resist the reward of sugary, fatty, salty treats: Your willpower has been gutted. The diet will tell you that it's your fault you regained all that weight—but any plan that expects you to change emotional attachments and physiological responses like pleasure, reward, and habit through sheer willpower is doomed from the start.

Diets also don't address your habits or your relationship with food, only your current intake. They don't teach you how to reward yourself in different ways, how to untangle your emotional ties to food, how to build healthy food habits (or break existing bad habits), or how to change your tastes to favor fresh, nutritious food. In fact, most encourage pre-packaged meals, bars, shakes, or powders, all of which move you even further away from a healthy relationship with food.

Finally, most quick-fix diets offer little to no structured support, motivation, or accountability while you're on the program—just a list of "Dos and Don'ts"—and no preparation for reentering the real world when the diet is over. But they'll promise you *this* is the one that will work, and you'll never have to diet ever again—as if once you lose 10 pounds, your tastes, dietary habits, and emotional relationship with food will be so completely transformed that you'll never go back to the foods you've been eating for decades: the same highly rewarding, comforting, familiar foods that made you overweight and unhealthy in the first place.

It must be magic.

So if the first step toward food freedom isn't a diet, what is it?

It's called a reset.

Push the reset button with your health, habits, and relationship with food, wipe the slate clean, and create a new foundation on which to build the perfect balanced, sustainable, healthy diet for *you*.

Now, maybe that sounds a little intimidating. We can all figure out how to diet (cut calories; restrict carbs or fat; replace meals with pills, powders, or shakes) in an effort to lose some weight. But designing a true dietary reset, one that reconnects you with your body, frees you from overpowering cravings, puts you in control of the food you eat, and leaves you feeling better than you have in years (or maybe *ever*)?

Yeah, that's hard.

RESET VS. DIET

How does a reset differ from a diet? First, a reset focuses on improving your overall health, not just on losing weight. Second, it encourages the formation of new habits, overwriting the old unhealthy habits that got you into trouble in the first place. Third, it helps you address and redefine your relationship with food, and find other ways to reward or comfort yourself and relieve stress. Finally, a true "reset" will change your physiology (your taste buds, blood sugar regulation, energy regulation, hormonal balance, digestion, and immune system) such that your new healthy habits are supported from the inside out.

CHAPTER 4

THE RESET (ELIMINATION)

Welcome to the first step in the
Food Freedom plan: a reset of your health,
habits, and relationship with food.

STEP 1:
THE RESET

- Completely eliminate foods that may have a negative impact.
- Note what changes.
- Reintroduce foods carefully and systematically.*
- Note what changes.

This process will be covered in detail in chapter 5.

Your first decision in Step 1 is choosing a reset that works for you. You'll have plenty of options; I'll outline several reset templates (including the Whole30), and give you all the information you'll need to design your own reset based on your specific context and goals.

When considering which reset to follow, I encourage you to factor these into your decision:

DO YOU ALREADY HAVE DIETARY RESTRICTIONS? If you're staunchly vegan or have multiple fruit, vegetable, or protein allergies, you'll want your reset to accommodate those restrictions in a healthy, manageable way.

HOW MUCH STRUCTURE DO YOU NEED? Some of you want a detailed, proven plan to follow. ("Tell me exactly what to do and I'll do it.") Others want to be more self-directed and fluid in their plan. ("Give me all the information and let me figure it out myself.") Think about how much heavy lifting you are able to do based on your day-to-day obligations, emotional state, and stress levels.

WHAT CAMP DO YOU FALL INTO? Back in chapter 2, I described readers as falling into one of two categories: those who feel truly powerless over food, and those who are simply looking to improve their health, habits, and relationship with food. The more serious you are in your quest for food freedom, the more aggressive I'll ask you to be with the elimination portion of your reset.

WHAT ARE YOUR MAIN GOALS? If you're here specifically to conquer your Sugar Dragon, your reset will look a little different than that of someone hoping to pinpoint the source of their digestive distress or joint pain.

DO YOU HAVE A MEDICAL CONDITION? As I'll explain on page 32, these resets are not designed to be stand-alone medical elimination diets, but many (like the Whole30) can be incredibly effective at identifying food sensitivities and resolving symptoms. Work closely with your health care practitioner to decide which reset is best.

Implementing an effective reset is the very foundation of food freedom, which is why this chapter is a hefty one. Keep the above questions in mind when reviewing your options, and know that no matter which reset you choose, it will start you down the path of lasting food freedom. However, I'm going to both reveal my bias and try to make this step really easy right now.

Let's talk about the Whole30.

Reset Option 1: The Whole30

The Whole30 was designed to help you figure out which foods are less healthy for *you*, then teach you how to use that information to create your own ideal, sustainable, balanced diet, because there is no one-size-fits-all. If you choose Whole30 as your reset, you will find that much of the heavy lifting of Step 1 has been done for you.

The Whole30 is not a diet: It's the catalyst for a whole new lifestyle. It's focused on health, not weight loss. In fact, you're not even allowed to step on the scale for the duration of the program, giving you a welcome, well-deserved respite from any obsession with body weight, and freeing you up to observe and appreciate all the benefits in so many areas of your life.

There is no calorie restriction. You will never be hungry.

There is no counting, measuring, or tracking your food. You'll have basic portion guidelines, but the program's structure gets you back in touch with your body's own regulatory signals to help you figure out how much to eat, and how to differentiate between cravings and true hunger.

Start to finish, the Whole30 reset is designed to create new, healthy habits while helping you become aware of, evaluate, and change your relationship with food. Lessons from habit and willpower research are built right into the program, because nothing changes in the long term until you actively work to create new patterns of behavior and understand the reasons behind your less healthy food choices. The Whole30 even helps you change your tastes, so by the end of the program you'll have a new appreciation for the delicious flavors of fresh, natural foods.

THE WHOLE30, IN A NUTSHELL

Here's how the Whole30 works: For a full 30 days, you completely eliminate the foods that the scientific literature and our clinical experience have deemed to be the most commonly problematic in one of four areas—your cravings, metabolism, digestion, and immune system. During the elimination period, you'll be completely avoiding these foods for a set period of time, experiencing what life is like without these commonly problematic triggers while paying careful attention to improvements in energy, sleep, digestion, mood, attention span, self-confidence, cravings, chronic pain or fatigue, athletic performance and recovery, and any number of other symptoms or medical conditions. This elimination period will give you a new "normal": a healthy baseline where, in all likelihood, you will look, feel, and live better than you ever imagined you could. At the end of the 30 days, you then carefully and systematically reintroduce those foods you've been missing, again paying attention to any changes in your experience. Do your 2 p.m. energy slumps return? Is your stomach bloated? Does your face break out, do your joints swell, does your pain return? Is your Sugar Dragon rearing his ugly head? The reintroduction period teaches you how specific foods are having a negative impact on *you* and exactly how these foods are making you look and feel less than your best. Put it all together, and for the first time in your life, you'll be able to make educated decisions about when, how often, and in what amount you can include these "less healthy" foods in your daily diet in a way that feels balanced and sustainable, but still keeps you feeling as awesome as you now *know* you can feel.

Most Whole30ers report that by the end of their program, their old treats (especially soda, fast food, junk food, and things with artificial sweeteners) are less enjoyable, making it easy to say "no." Sometimes laughably so: Whole30er Diana B. says, "After our Whole30 was over, my husband and I were in town one night doing some errands. We were starving and unprepared and decided to whip into our pre-Whole30 favorite fast-food place. We got our standard orders, took a few bites, looked at each other with amazement, and were like, 'Gah, how did we ever think this stuff was good?'"

The Whole30 also comes with a robust support network (a daily e-mail service during your program; a free forum staffed by Whole30 experts; and a friendly, helpful, and extremely active social media community) designed to keep you motivated, hold you accountable, and help you maximize your success. Finally, this book was specifically designed to mesh seamlessly with the Whole30, and includes all the tools you will need to maintain your food freedom long after the 30 days are over.

"EVERYTHING IN MODERATION"

Some people don't understand the need for a reset, especially one as structured as the Whole30. These are the people who ask, "Why can't you just eat everything in moderation?" (Bless their hearts.) That's nice in theory . . . but if that concept actually worked for most people, we'd all be happy, healthy, lean, and fit, because we've all been trying to moderate for decades. The truth is that most people just *can't* moderate when it comes to highly rewarding, low-satiety foods in the context of their busy, stressful lives. Once you're stuck in the cycle of craving → overconsumption → guilt and shame → stress → more cravings, you can't recalibrate your taste buds, hormones, digestive tract, and immune system without a major overhaul—a short-term "rehab" for your body and brain. It sounds like a drastic measure, especially to the select few who are able to successfully moderate, but for the oh-so-many who can't, the idea of a structured, supported reset where someone else makes the hard food decisions for you until you're back on track actually sounds like heaven, not deprivation.

The Whole30 Reset Rules

Here are the basics of the Whole30 program, but I recommend you read *The Whole30: The 30-Day Guide to Total Health and Food Freedom* for a complete list of rules, and use that book to prepare for and succeed with your reset. (Bonus: It also features more than 100 delicious Whole30-compliant recipes.)

For the next 30 days, you'll be eating meat, seafood, and eggs; lots of vegetables and fruit; and natural, healthy fats—with no slips, cheats, or special occasions. At the same time, you'll be eliminating a host of ingredients. Brace yourself: The list is not for the faint of heart and probably includes a whole bunch of foods you really like. But as the most-quoted line of the Whole30 goes, "Beating cancer is hard. Birthing a baby is hard. Losing a parent is hard. Drinking your coffee black. Is. Not. Hard." You've done harder things than this, and it's for the best cause on earth: the only physical body you will ever have in this lifetime.

Remember, it's only 30 days.

DO NOT CONSUME ADDED SUGAR OF ANY KIND, REAL OR ARTIFICIAL. No maple syrup, honey, agave nectar, coconut sugar, Splenda, Equal, Nutrasweet, xylitol, stevia, etc. Read your labels, because companies sneak sugar into products in ways you might not recognize.

DO NOT CONSUME ALCOHOL IN ANY FORM. No wine, beer, champagne, vodka, rum, whiskey, tequila, etc., whether drunk on its own or used as an ingredient—not even for cooking.

DO NOT EAT GRAINS. This includes wheat, rye, barley, oats, corn, rice, millet, bulgur, sorghum, sprouted grains, and all gluten-free pseudo-cereals like amaranth, buckwheat, or quinoa. This also includes all the ways we add wheat, corn, and rice into our foods in the form of bran, germ, starch, and so on. Again, read your labels.

DO NOT EAT LEGUMES. This includes beans of all kinds (black, red, pinto, navy, white, kidney, lima, fava, etc.), peas, chickpeas, lentils, and peanuts. This also includes all forms of soy—soy sauce, miso, tofu, tempeh, edamame, and all the ways we sneak soy into foods (like soybean oil or soy lecithin). No peanut butter, either. The only exceptions are green beans and snow peas or snap peas.

DO NOT EAT DAIRY. This includes cow's-, goat's-, or sheep's-milk products such as cream, cheese, kefir, yogurt, and sour cream. The only exceptions are clarified butter and ghee.

DO NOT CONSUME CARRAGEENAN, MSG, OR ADDED SULFITES. If these ingredients appear in any form in the ingredient list of your processed food or beverage, it's out for the Whole30.

DO NOT RECREATE BAKED GOODS, "TREATS," OR JUNK FOODS WITH APPROVED INGREDIENTS. No banana-egg pancakes, Paleo bread, or coconut milk ice cream. (See the box below for more details.) Your cravings and habits won't change if you keep eating these foods, even if they are made with Whole30 ingredients.

DO NOT STEP ON THE SCALE OR TAKE MEASUREMENTS. Your reset is about so much more than just weight loss; focusing on your body composition means you'll miss out on the most dramatic and lifelong benefits this plan has to offer. Feel free to take before-and-after measurements, but no weighing yourself, analyzing body fat, or breaking out the tape measure during your Whole30.

LET'S GET SPECIFIC

A few off-limits foods that fall under the "No baked goods, treats, or recreated junk foods" rule include: pancakes, bread, tortillas, biscuits, crepes, muffins, cupcakes, cookies, pizza crust, waffles, cereal, potato chips, French fries, and that one recipe where eggs, date paste, and coconut milk are combined with prayers to create a thick, creamy concoction that can once again transform your undrinkable black coffee into sweet, dreamy caffeine. However, while this list of off-limits foods applies to everyone (even those who don't "have a problem" with bread or pancakes), you may decide your personal Off-Limits List includes additional foods which you already know make you feel out of control. (See page 95 in *The Whole30* for guidance.)

You, on the Whole30 Reset

Now that you've had a preview of the Whole30 and its rules, here's how your journey on the Whole30 reset will look. (Feel free to compare it to the grim recap of your previous dieting experiences.)

You prepare for the program using our extensive resources and feedback from the Whole30 community, feeling supported through the entire process. You understand why the program rules are specifically designed in this manner, and you've connected with one or more of the emotional, psychological, or physical benefits of the program, giving you internal motivation (far stronger than "beach weather is coming") to see it through.

You still need willpower to resist surprise temptations, but because the rules are so clearly defined and you're supporting your commitment from the inside out (with a resetting of your taste buds, hormones, digestion, and immune system), you'll need to call on it far less. Using the community's resources and guidance, you've also created detailed plans for dealing with stressful situations, making it far less likely you'll cave in to pressure in the moment.

During your 30 days, you're in tune with what's changing in your body and your brain every step of the way because you're free from the shackles of the scale. You create new, healthy habits and discover other ways to reward yourself, comfort yourself, and share love with others. You don't have to count calories or track your intake, which fosters a healthy relationship with food and meal times. You're never hungry and are eating lots of vitamins, minerals, and other nutrients, which makes your cravings less powerful and keeps your metabolism humming. Your tastes change, your cravings dissipate, and you discover new foods to love.

You relearn how to listen to your body, sleep better, have more energy, and feel more confident. You successfully change your life (and you may have to buy new clothes in a smaller size). You are able to create your own perfect healthy eating plan based on what you've learned from your Whole30 reintroduction. You lose the idea of food being good or bad; there is no more guilt or shame, only choices and consequences.

You stay close to the Whole30 community once you're back in the "real world," living your new, healthy habits, and come back to the program for a reset when you find yourself drifting back toward less healthy behaviors. You could do this forever and be optimally healthy ... but eventually, you won't need to return to the program because you'll effortlessly be making smart food decisions for yourself, and your new healthy habits will be so ingrained that you'll no longer need to reset at all.

THIS is food freedom.

Sounds way better, right?

READY TO TRY THE WHOLE30?

I f you're open to the idea of using the Whole30 as your reset, this makes your Food Freedom plan so much easier. Still need a little more encouragement? First, the Whole30 program has been endorsed by a number of respected dietitians, medical doctors, and psychiatrists, and many medical professionals are using the program with their patients with great success. Second, you'll be incredibly supported using the extensive resources provided; no need to create your own meal plans, shopping lists, or recipes. Third, hundreds of thousands of people have already testified to the program's life-changing effects. Finally, *it's only 30 days*, and committing to the Whole30 now means you're well on your way to completing Step 1 of this Food Freedom plan. If you're in, just follow the program as outlined in *The Whole30* and return to this book after your reintroduction, when you're ready to move on to Step 2: Enjoying Your Food Freedom (see chapter 6). If you're still not sold and want to continue by building your own reset, roll up your sleeves—there's work to be done.

Reset Option 2: Design Your Own

For a number of reasons, the Whole30 may not be the right reset for you. If you have your own self-imposed dietary restrictions (like no animal products), need less rigidity, or don't think you're ready to take on a change as dramatic as the Whole30, you can still craft an effective reset using the tools in this book.

Even if you intend to create your own reset, there are still concepts you can pull from the Whole30—and you should, as these have proven critical to the success of individuals on the program.

First and most important, focus on *health*, not weight loss. Regardless of the foods you choose to eat on your reset, your goal is to improve your physical, psychological, and emotional health. (Get that straight, and body composition will naturally follow.) Besides, trying to lose weight fast is what got you into trouble in the first place, isn't it? So let's do something different here.

To that extent, I recommend banishing the scale and not taking measurements for the duration of your program, just as required on the Whole30. Free yourself from the preoccupation with body weight and allow yourself the space to focus on all the other things that are changing as the result of your healthy eating efforts.

Next, craft your reset to include an elimination and reintroduction period, just like the Whole30. *This is mandatory.* Get rid of the ingredients you think may be having a negative impact on your health, habits, and relationship with food, and evaluate what life is like without those potentially problematic foods. Then, very carefully and systematically, reintroduce the items you've been missing, one at a time, so you can evaluate the impact of bringing them back.

MEDICAL CONDITIONS

I t's important to note that neither the Whole30 nor any of the sample reset plans outlined in this chapter are designed to be *medical elimination diets*. They weren't created to help you treat any specific medical condition and aren't a substitute for working with a trained health-care practitioner. If you have a chronic disease or condition that requires a more serious health intervention than a self-designed reset, you have two options. The first, with your health-care practitioner's blessing, is to try the Whole30 reset as outlined. The program excludes most of the food groups a medical doctor would as part of a standard elimination, and the feedback gathered during the reintroduction phase can help you determine if you're on the right track. The second option is to work directly with a functional medicine* or other trained health-care provider to create an elimination diet designed specifically for your context and medical condition.

*Functional medicine is a patient-centered practice in which a provider takes your unique genetic, environmental, and biochemical factors into consideration and strives to treat your mind, body, and spirit as a whole. These practitioners are particularly interested in addressing your nutrition, stress levels, and toxin exposure in an effort to prevent and treat chronic disease. For more information, go to page 235.

This is how you can identify which foods make *you* less healthy. Without elimination and careful reintroduction, you won't learn nearly as much from your reset as you could, and it will be next to impossible to craft the perfect, sustainable diet for yourself moving forward.

NON-SCALE VICTORIES

The list of potential victories you could achieve with your reset is long, and it includes a fafillion wins that have nothing to do with the scale: Fewer blemishes. Thicker hair. Less joint pain. Reduced cravings. No midday energy slump. A sunnier disposition. At Whole30, we call these types of improvements "non-scale victories" (#NSV on social media). You can download a Non-Scale Victory checklist with more than 100 NSVs at w30.co/whole30nsv; use it at the start of your reset to highlight areas in which you'd like to see improvement. Post it in a visible spot and check in with it throughout your reset to keep your motivation high and help you identify the areas of your life that are changing as a result of your efforts. At the end of your reset, go back and check off all the things that you have accomplished. Be generous here! You've worked hard, and small victories are still victories (and a sign that your reset was effective).

Elimination

An elimination diet is a procedure used to identify and exclude foods that may be causing an adverse effect in a person, after which those foods are reintroduced one at a time. Often-problematic foods that tend to be excluded as part of an elimination diet (in part or all at once) include gluten-containing grains (wheat, barley and rye), gluten-free grains (like corn or oats), dairy, added sugar, artificial sweeteners, food dyes, sulfites, eggs, peanuts, soy, legumes (beans, peas, lentils), citrus fruits, beef, caffeine, alcohol, nuts and seeds, nightshade vegetables (such as tomatoes, eggplant, white potatoes, and peppers), and foods high in FODMAPs (fermentable carbohydrates that can promote digestive distress in sensitive individuals). You may also choose to exclude foods that you simply suspect don't work for you—for example, ingredients you already know you're allergic to, or foods that commonly give you digestive or skin issues.

It's important to frame these often-problematic foods in the right context. In fact, how you choose to think about them during the elimination phase of your reset can profoundly influence what happens when you choose to reintroduce them. Big picture, keep this one thing in mind:

These foods are not inherently "bad" or "unhealthy."

While the scientific literature suggests that many of these foods are commonly problematic to some degree for a broad range of people, *that doesn't make them bad for everyone.* Nearly every single one of the foods you'll eliminate during your reset contains both health-promoting (whether it's physical or psychological) *and* health-degrading potential. Milk contains valuable minerals, but also includes carbohydrates that may disrupt digestion. Whole grains have fiber, but may provoke an immune response. Some studies show that drinking alcohol (in the right amounts and the right context) can actually be health-promoting. Someone who struggles to digest broccoli would vehemently disagree if I were to proclaim that broccoli is good for everyone. You simply cannot make a blanket statement about any food being "healthy" or "unhealthy," despite what the news headlines often scream.

Repeat after me: These foods aren't "good" or "bad," they're just "unknown." I'm spelling this out now because later, when you reintroduce them into your diet, this will help you skip the part where you feel guilty about bringing "bad" stuff back into your new, healthy lifestyle. (Just in case, I'll remind you again on page 61.)

The more foods you exclude, the better chance you have of identifying sensitivities . . . but the harder the diet is to follow, especially since the key to an elimination diet is the *complete removal* of suspect foods during the elimination period. Like, *complete.* No bite of a friend's coffee cake, no splash of milk in your coffee, no "just this once" glass of wine. No.

Say you live with a number of pets: five cats. Every day, your nose is a little itchy, your eyes are a little red, and your throat is scratchy. You love all your cats, but you recognize that you don't feel well, and you'd like to feel better. You start to wonder if one of your cats is the culprit.

So in an effort to figure out your sensitivities, you send four cats to your mom's house for a month. But you keep one cat, because he barely ever comes inside, and one tiny snuggle with your cat once in a while probably won't hurt. (Plus, some days are stressful, and you really *need* your cat to help you unwind.)

Do you feel better? Maybe, kind of. Are you able to compare how you feel in a cat-free environment to how you feel when your cats are around? Nope. Do you know whether it's the animals at all, or maybe just the fact that you haven't dusted in a year? Uh, nope. The need for *total* elimination of potentially problematic pets should be obvious by now . . . and it's no different with your bread, wine, cheese, cookies, and peanut butter.

Find something else to snuggle after a hard day at the office. Like your spouse, a good book, or a cutting board. (I actually find chopping vegetables to be very therapeutic.)

Finally, design your reset based on your capacity for sticking to it, but try to "go big"—as broad you can, eliminating as many potentially problematic foods as possible. Remember, your reset is just a short-term experiment, not your lifelong dietary plan, so you should learn as much as you possibly can from the experience. The more foods you eliminate, the more opportunity you'll have to learn how food has been impacting you during reintroduction, which means your perfect food freedom diet will be that much more specifically tailored to your goals and context.

STRUCTURED ELIMINATION DIETS

A number of elimination protocols exist, including the Paleo Autoimmune Protocol (AIP), for those with diagnosed autoimmune conditions; the Specific Carbohydrate Diet (SCD), designed to naturally treat chronic inflammatory conditions in the digestive tract; the Gut and Psychology Syndrome (GAPS) diet, a derivative of the SCD designed to treat a variety of intestinal and neurological conditions; low-FODMAP diets, which eliminate foods high in fermentable carbohydrates to improve IBS (Irritable Bowel Syndrome) and other digestive conditions; and other protocols designed for those with a specific medical condition or health concern. However, these protocols are even *more* restrictive than the Whole30, and more complicated to follow. Still, if you really want to go big with the elimination phase of your reset, you can consult the resources on page 236 to adopt one of these more stringent but well-defined protocols.

Now that we're in agreement that a health-focused elimination and reintroduction are the very foundation of a reset, all that's left to decide is what, specifically, you'll be eliminating.

Planning Your Elimination

Let's outline the general structure of your reset before we get into the specifics of the foods you'll be eliminating. First, the duration of the elimination period should be between 30 and 60 days—perhaps in certain circumstances longer, but certainly no less. The "30" in Whole30 comes from habit research that suggests it takes, on average, 66 days for a new habit to stick.* However, when you're talking about changing something as emotional as your diet, the idea of a two-month intervention is intimidating. You don't want your reset to be so long that it seems unrealistic to accomplish, but it has to be long enough to see results and make progress in creating new, healthy habits. Thirty days is a nice compromise; long enough to experience dramatic improvements in your health and relationship with food, but also attainable—most people say, "I can do anything for thirty days."

LONGER THAN 30?

If you have a chronic condition (like eczema, fatigue, or pain), an autoimmune disease, or sugar addiction, you may require a longer intervention for symptoms to improve. Feel free to choose a longer duration for your elimination, or start with 30 days and decide if you want to keep going as Day 30 nears, based on how well you've responded and your comfort with continuing. Note that I don't recommend going any longer than 90 days without taking a break to evaluate how well it's working and seeing how your body responds to the reintroduction of foods you've been missing. Remember, food freedom demands that you make your own decisions—and it's hard to do that if you're blindly following your reset rules all the time, turning down special or delicious "off-plan" food that may actually be worth it. That's not true freedom—that's self-imposed house arrest, even if you are pretty satisfied with your reset diet.

Second, your reset should be centered around real, whole, nutrient-dense foods, avoiding all refined food-like products. Real foods the way nature designed them—with complete protein, natural fats, fiber, water, and micronutrients—contain built-in satiety factors, helping you get back

---

* The common belief that it takes 21 days to make or break a habit came from a surgeon's observations taken out of context in the 1950s; like a game of telephone, the misrepresentation of his conclusions morphed into the idea that new habits can be fully formed in just three weeks. However, recent studies show that 21 days falls grossly short of the time it actually takes to change something as emotional as your diet—in fact, with some initiatives (like quitting smoking), it may take as long as eight months for new habits to really take hold.

in touch with your body's "hungry" and "full" signals, reducing cravings, making you less likely to snack on sweets between meals, and resensitizing your taste buds to appreciate the delicious flavors found in fresh foods.

This means opting for whole, unprocessed foods ahead of shakes or smoothies; cooking your own organic tofu-veggie stir-fry instead of choosing a processed veggie burger; and avoiding technically-compliant-but-not-in-the-spirit-of-a-reset sweets, treats, and baked goods. That means no vegan chocolate cupcakes, grain-free cookies, or almond-flour tortillas, even if the ingredients technically fit your plan.

That last bit is wildly unpopular, but also for your own good.

How are you supposed to execute an effective reset of your habits and emotional relationship with food if you're still eating waffles, cookies, and bread? Your brain doesn't know the difference between an almond-flour pancake and a "real" pancake ... it just knows it's still getting pancakes. If one of your goals is to break your reliance on sweets and treats, *you can't keep eating them.*

This is a nonnegotiable part of your reset. Without it, the Food Freedom program looks like any other diet that allows you to retain your bad habits and reliance on sweets while still remaining *technically* compliant. That approach does not lead to lasting results. That approach will not bring you food freedom. That approach keeps you stuck in the same place with the same cravings and the same bad habits, but you don't even realize it because you're still giving yourself a gold star for following "the plan."

It's not your fault. The plan is bad. So we're not going to repeat the same mistakes with our reset. NO PANCAKES, #sorrynotsorry.

Next, your reset must exclude all alcohol. Do I really need to explain how alcohol is hindering your progress toward getting healthy (and losing weight), preventing you from learning how to reward or comfort yourself in a healthier way, and causing you to make poor food choices? Alcohol shouldn't play a role in *any* health-focused reset, regardless of the specific foods you choose to eat. Remember, it's only 30 days. Also, if you're getting all kinds of defensive at the idea of going without wine for 30 days, I'm going to invite you evaluate your relationship with wine and suggest that 30 days without it is probably exactly what you need. (See "No pancakes.")

Your reset should also exclude all forms of added sugar or artificial sweeteners, just like the Whole30. That means if there is any sort of sugar—even the stuff that seems natural and maybe even good for you, like honey, agave, or stevia—or artificial sweeteners in the ingredient list, it's out for your reset. (This doesn't include foods with organically occurring sugars, like fruit or sweet potatoes—it only applies to *added* sugar.) This also means no sugar in your coffee, honey in your tea, or Splenda over your strawberries, which may sound strange, but I know for a fact that some of you think your strawberries don't taste sweet without it.

If that's your context, I'm glad you're here.

Now, some of you may be thinking, "My sugar habit isn't *that* serious. I don't really need to go *that* far. A little sugar here and there isn't *that* big of a deal." Trust me: It doesn't have to be . . . and you actually do . . . and it actually is.

POUR SOME SUGAR ON ME

According to the Center for Science in the Public Interest, the average American consumes about 23 teaspoons of sugar a day. That's *78 pounds a year, per person,* from foods like soda, candy, energy drinks, and desserts—stuff we know we should be avoiding. But there are also significant amounts of added sugar in "healthy" foods like soup, deli meat, almond milk, tomato sauce, single-serving coffee packets, protein bars, dried fruit, and condiments—and unless you're reading every label and making a conscious decision to skip *any* food with added sugar, they'll start piling up. It's going to be frustrating once you realize there's sugar in *everything,* but Whole30ers report that label-reading and avoiding added sugar is a habit that has stuck with them long after their reset ended, reinforcing their new healthy habits and the growth mind-set (see page 104) they achieved during the program.

There are a few benefits to this "no added sugar" rule. First, it makes decisions easy. Just read your labels: If there's added sugar, it's out—no deliberation or willpower required. Second, it creates a habit of looking at what's in your food, which allows you to make educated decisions about what you eat. Third, sugar is what makes people feel most out of control. Eliminating all sources of added sugar provides the perfect reset environment for your taste buds and brain. By not allowing any wiggle room, you won't try to justify eating "just one" sweet treat along the way. Finally, adopting this rule will help you stick to "no baked goods or junk foods," because nearly all those products contain added sugar.

Seriously, you should do this.

Finally, make your reset as "black and white" as possible. This approach gets a bad rap from people who see it as being overly restrictive (see the box on page 40), but habit research proves that black-and-white rules are actually easier for the brain to follow, moving the decision-making process out of "effort" territory into "habit" territory. Set clear expectations for what you will and will not be eating, and make the rules nonnegotiable. The clearer you can make your reset guidelines, the easier it will be to stick to the program, and the less willpower you'll require to stay compliant.

Avoid using fuzzy terms like "less," "more," or "better" ("I'll eat less cheese"; "I'll be better about watching my sugar intake"). These are hard for the brain to interpret, and require more energy and willpower to execute as the brain struggles to decide "Less than what?" or "Is this better?" Instead, use definitive words like "no" or "only" or "always." Instead of "I'll eat more vegetables," say, "I'll avoid all grains, and replace them only with vegetables and fruit." Instead of "I'll drink less wine," say, "No alcohol in any form, not even for cooking."

Ideally, this black-and-white approach includes initiating a "No cheats, no slips, no excuses" rule for your reset period, just like the Whole30. Unless you have a history of disordered eating* (for which this kind of rigidity can be triggering), you need to fully commit to the plan, removing any opportunity for your brain to stage a rebellion in which it encourages you to treat yourself "just this once," thereby unraveling your reset.

Before moving on to the design of your reset, here's one final thing I want you to know: Designing the elimination portion is the trickiest part of the entire Food Freedom plan. It's a bit like shooting at a target while blindfolded, because you don't have scientific consensus *or* your own personal health practitioner's recommendations backing up your choices. In the next chapter, I'll talk about what happens if your reset isn't as effective as you may have hoped, but for now, know that if you're *not* doing the Whole30 or working with a health-care provider to design a custom reset, your self-designed plan may need some tweaks along the way (and/or require multiple attempts) before you find the protocol that's the most physically, psychologically, and emotionally successful for you.

Now that you understand the why and how behind the elimination phase, it's time to decide which reset is right for you. After that's settled, I'll go into detail about the second (and equally important) phase of your reset: reintroduction.

---

* If you currently suffer from an eating disorder or have a history of disordered eating, you *must* work with a trained counselor or health-care practitioner to design a reset approach that is appropriate for your unique context.

ISN'T THIS *TOO* RESTRICTIVE?

Some critics of the Whole30's "all or nothing" approach suggest the rigidity of the rules is unhealthy, and that this kind of deprivation only leads to a rebound once the program is over. With many super-restrictive diets, this would be valid criticism—but with your reset, it's wholly unfounded. First, you're not restricting calories or nutrients, so you're never stressed with hunger. (You're also not counting, weighing, measuring, or tracking your food, which eliminates a whole lot of anxiety around mealtime.) Second, these black-and-white rules are designed to take some of the burden of decision-making out of your hands, so you're relying less on willpower and self-regulation and feeling more in control of your food (which is actually freeing, not restrictive). Finally, remember: It's only 30 days. You aren't going to have rigid rules like this forever—just during the elimination period, where it's mission-critical to stay compliant.

Sample Resets

With the basic rules out of the way, it's time to really dial in on the specific foods you'll be eliminating for the next few weeks, based on your goals. I'll provide some general reset examples based on both my clinical experience (having observed thousands of people go through the Whole30 program) and the current scientific consensus on the most commonly problematic foods.

I can't choose your reset for you. Here's where you'll need to step in and take over.

From the long list of potential foods/food groups on page 41, figure out how "big" you can go; how many of these potentially problematic items you're willing to completely eliminate for the duration of your program. While deciding, take into account how these foods have impacted you in the past; not just physically, but psychologically and emotionally. If there are any standouts (dairy always gives me gas), target them immediately. If there's anything here that's easy (I don't eat soy anyway), eliminate those foods by default. If there's one thing on this list that makes you say, "Not that—I *cannot* live without that," it should absolutely, positively be eliminated.

You hate that, I know, but it's for your own good. That food is your kryptonite, and you've gotta stash it far, far away during your reset.

Then, from the rest, craft a detailed list of your "off-limits" foods, making it as broad as possible.

- Gluten-containing grains
- Gluten-free grains
- Dairy
- Added sugar
- Artificial sweeteners
- Food dyes
- Sulfites
- Eggs
- Peanuts
- Soy
- Legumes
- Citrus fruits
- Beef
- Caffeine
- Alcohol
- Nuts and seeds
- Nightshades (see page 46)
- High-FODMAP foods (see page 50)

At the absolute bare minimum, you need to eliminate all forms of gluten, dairy, and alcohol, consuming minimally processed foods and beverages and avoiding added sugar and artificial sweeteners. From there, you can tailor your reset according to your specific health mission. Read on for five plans that have been customized according to some of the most common reset goals: eliminating cravings, reducing inflammation, restoring energy, accommodating a vegan framework, and resetting with less specific goals in mind or a reduced capacity for change.

READ. EVERY. LABEL.

Ideally, most of your reset foods won't even have a label, because you'll be basing your reset diet on whole, unprocessed foods. Still, you'll also be buying condiments, pantry staples, dressings, and beverages, and if this is all new to you, I'll warn you up front: Avoiding things like gluten and dairy is harder than it sounds. Gluten is hidden in *lots* of things (soup, sauces, spices, even tea), and dairy may take cover under a variety of names (like whey or casein) on the nutritional label. The key to complete avoidance is educating yourself on the hidden forms of these foods (visit whole30.com/pdf-downloads for resources) and reading *every single label* during the elimination period. It sounds exhausting, but you'll quickly become skilled at recognizing off-plan ingredients, and once you identify the brand of broth/tomato sauce/almond milk that fits your reset, you won't have to go through the trouble of reading ten labels just to find one that works. Be vigilant here. Remember, 100% compliance is key, and if it turns out you're sensitive, even tiny amounts of these off-plan ingredients could break some physiological aspects of your "reset" (namely, healing the gut and calming the immune system).

CRAVING-BUSTER RESET

On this reset, you'll be completely eliminating the following foods and beverages:

- Grains
- Dairy
- Nuts, seeds, or dried fruit
- Alcohol
- Added sugar
- Artificial sweeteners
- Sweets/treats/baked goods

Taming your Sugar Dragon starts with eliminating all forms of grains. That means no bread, corn tortillas, oatmeal, or other carb-dense comfort foods you're used to relying on. This rule will also help you stay away from technically compliant sweets, treats, and baked goods..

You're also not eating any dairy. That means no cheese. You don't like this. It's still for your own good.

YOU HEART CHEESE.

Over the course of more than 100 nutrition seminars, I asked attendees, "If I told you that you could never eat dairy ever again, what's the one food you'd miss the most?" In every single seminar but one, the participants agreed their most beloved dairy product was cheese. (Huntsville, Alabama, said ice cream.) In fact, in a recent discussion on social media, the vast majority of respondents said they are just as likely to comfort-binge on cheese as on grain-based snack foods! Brandy B. said, "Cheese is a major emotional trigger food . . . eliminating cheese is some serious dragon-slaying for me." And Andrea V. made a great point about the foods you probably eat cheese with: "I used to eat huge cheese plates, paired with nuts, honey, and wine. Cheese is addictive for me." If you're *that* dependent on the stuff, you know it's gotta come out for your reset, right?

There's another reason dairy is out for the Craving-Buster reset: You may think of dairy as "health food," but you'd be surprised how much sugar is in low-fat yogurt or flavored coffee creamers. (And do we even have to talk about ice cream and frozen yogurt?) My point is this: Not all craving-promoting foods have chocolate or flour in them. For 30 days, get your calcium and other bone-health-promoting micronutrients from fresh vegetables, meat, and seafood, because it's worth evaluating the role of dairy in your cravings.

In this plan, you're still omitting all forms of added sugar, artificial sweeteners, and alcohol (for obvious reasons), but you're also taking out two food groups that are generally considered healthy: nuts and seeds, and dried fruit. This is because your reward-driven, sugar-obsessed brain will try to play tricks on you. In the absence of the highly rewarding foods you used to eat (and still desperately crave), the brain will settle for whatever it can get. It can't have a candy bar, so it will direct you to a dried-fruit-and-nut bar. It can't have frosting or Nutella, so it will encourage you to eat almond butter by the spoonful. These are technically healthier food choices, but your brain doesn't know the difference. All your brain knows is, "I craved a reward . . . and I got it," which is not helping your craving-busting cause.

It's also easy overeat these foods (nuts and seeds are the perfect trifecta of salty, fatty, and crunchy; and dried fruit is basically nature's candy), which will keep you feeling out of control and a slave to your Sugar Dragon. And I won't even mention these foods in combination, like dates stuffed with almond butter.

Just no.

Finally, during your reset, remember to keep this previously mentioned question in mind: "Is eating this food in this moment actually helping me change my cravings?" If you're eating frozen grapes by the handful because you're dying for sugar, the answer is no. If you're replacing your usual dessert with a bowl of berries, toasted coconut flakes, and almond milk every single night, the answer is no. This reset requires so much awareness around the emotional reasons why you choose to eat certain foods at certain times, but the payoff for that honest introspection is huge: true food freedom, and a snoozing Sugar Dragon when all is said and done.

ANTI-INFLAMMATORY RESET

On this reset, you'll be completely eliminating the following foods and beverages:

- Grains
- Legumes
- Dairy
- Eggs
- Nightshades
- Alcohol
- Added sugar
- Artificial sweeteners
- Sweets/treats/baked goods

The Whole30 is by design an anti-inflammatory diet, but if you want to take our program one step further in an effort to calm chronic or serious inflammation, you could also eliminate eggs and nightshade vegetables.

All the proposed elimination foods outlined in both the Whole30 as well as this reset have been shown in scientific literature to promote inflammation in sensitive populations, to varying degrees. It may not make immediate sense that the bread you eat is tied to your joint pain or migraines, but this reset is designed to help you connect those dots. From a science-y perspective, this inflammation generally starts in the gut, when these foods interact with the lining of your small intestine and create some degree of permeability (known as "leaky gut"). They can also improperly cross the gut barrier or disrupt the delicate balance of gut bacteria, triggering an immune response and promoting systemic inflammation.

WHAT IS CHRONIC SYSTEMIC INFLAMMATION?

Inflammation happens when the immune system mobilizes to protect from and repair injury, infection, or other damage to the body. Usually this response can be quite helpful, like when your body detects the influenza virus and sends out an army of white blood cells in an effort to mop it up. The inflammatory response was designed to help with short-term, specific issues like this. But thanks to less-than-healthy diet and lifestyle choices, more and more people are living with a chronic, systemic inflammatory response in which the immune system is fired up 24/7 throughout the entire body, creating all sorts of health issues. This kind of inflammation is at the root of a huge number of lifestyle-related diseases and conditions, including obesity, diabetes, heart disease, stroke, high cholesterol, autoimmune diseases like lupus or rheumatoid arthritis, and neurological conditions like Alzheimer's disease and Parkinson's disease. It also figures into day-to-day issues like tendinitis, asthma, allergies, acne, depression, and ADHD. The truth is, most people are inflamed to some degree. If you're overweight, you've got inflammation. If you suffer from a laundry list of nagging health issues (think: allergies, asthma, migraines, or eczema), you've got inflammation. If you're underslept, overstressed, or not eating enough micronutrients, you've got inflammation. And if you're experiencing tangible, serious signs (like joint pain and swelling, an autoimmune condition, or chronic fatigue or pain), inflammation is definitely at play. While there are multiple factors contributing to your health woes, the regular consumption of foods that impair the gut and upregulate the immune system is one of the biggest causative factors in systemic inflammation. The Anti-Inflammatory Reset will tackle that.

This reset also cuts out two specific food groups—nightshades and eggs—that have been shown to be extra problematic in certain individuals, especially those with joint issues or chronic medical conditions.

NIGHTSHADES

Nightshades are a group of plants that contain compounds that may be inflammatory in those who have a digestive sensitivity. This comprehensive but not exhaustive* list includes:

- Tomatoes
- Tamarillos
- Tomatillos
- Potatoes (but not sweet potatoes or yams)
- Eggplant
- Bell/sweet peppers
- Cape gooseberry. ground cherries, or golden berry
- Goji berries
- Hot peppers (such as chile peppers, jalapeños, serranos, and habaneros)
- Hot sauces (like Tabasco)
- Pepinos
- Pepper- or chile-based spices (such as black pepper, red pepper flakes, paprika, or cayenne)
- Pimentos
- Ashwagandha (an Ayurvedic herb)

*There are many too many varieties of peppers, tomatoes, eggplants, potatoes, and spices to list here. For a far more comprehensive list, see the AIP resources on page 237.

Yeah, it's a lot of stuff; you need to know what you're getting yourself into here. Still, if you're really struggling with inflammation and are ready to "go big" to see potentially huge benefits, this is an option worth considering.

Eggs, specifically the egg whites, are also commonly problematic and are often tied to skin issues like eczema, joint issues like arthritis, or a worsening of autoimmune-related symptoms. If you're ready to "go big" or already suspect that eggs aren't working well for you, it's a good idea to eliminate them.

Taking on this protocol means being even more careful with your label-reading, as nightshade spices (like black pepper) appear in a lot of foods. And with eggs off the table, you'll have to get creative with breakfast. Remember, you *can* eat a burger, salmon, or chicken soup at 7 a.m.—there's no rule that says your morning meal must include eggs.

RECIPES!

Going without eggs and mealtime staples like tomato sauce or black pepper may seem daunting, but there is a whole world of recipes available to you, thanks to the popularity of the Paleo AIP. While that protocol eliminates even more foods than outlined here, you can still look to AIP recipes as good sources of egg- and nightshade-free meals. There are even specific nightshade-free spice blends (like those offered by Primal Palate, primalpalate.com), helping you add flavor to your meals without the risk of provoking an inflammatory response. (Refer to the resources starting on page 236 for websites and cookbooks.)

ENERGY RESET

On this reset, you'll be completely eliminating the following foods and beverages:

- Grains
- Dairy
- Caffeine
- Alcohol
- Added sugar
- Artificial sweeteners
- Sweets/treats/baked goods

The key focus of an energy reset is to teach your body to become "fat-adapted": able to use fat as fuel. If you've been eating a Standard American Diet (SAD)—even a "healthy" one based on whole grains and low-fat dairy—you've trained your body to rely on sugar for energy. This means you have to eat every two hours or you get "hangry," that unpleasant-for-you-and-everyone-around-you combination of "hungry" and "angry."

Your body can run really well on fat, too, but you have to teach it to do that by not spoon-feeding it carbs and sugar all the time. Ruling out added sugar, alcohol, sweets, and baked goods makes sense . . . but so does ruling out all forms of grains. As wholesome as they may seem, a bowl of brown rice, gluten-free oatmeal, or a whole-grain bagel still provides lots of carbohydrates (which breaks down into sugar in the body), training your body to be reliant on sugar for energy and sending you down that familiar brain-foggy, hungry-every-two-hours path. It's the carb-dense, nutrient-poor breads, cereals, and 100-calorie snack packs that got you into energy trouble in the first place, so we have to pull those out to let your mitochondria (your cellular "powerhouses") learn to use the fat from your body and your food for energy. That means subbing those grain-based carbs with nutrient-dense vegetables and fruit, and giving your body more healthy fats to run on.

You'll also want to eliminate dairy here, as it's often accompanied by lots of sugar and is so commonly problematic in the gut. Anything that disrupts the integrity of your digestive tract will also affect your energy levels, so let's rule that out by eliminating dairy during your reset.

Finally, caffeine. Oh, sweet coffee, the only thing that gets you out of bed in the morning (and your head off your desk mid-afternoon). If the main reason you're coming to a reset is to give your energy a boost, you'll need to do the one thing you desperately don't want to do: say bye-bye to coffee. (And energy drinks, and black tea, and soda . . .)

Before you panic, please remember one thing:

It's just a short-term experiment.

I'm not saying you can never have caffeine ever again. What I *am* saying is that you've been so reliant on caffeine to prop up your energy levels that you have no idea how to function without it—and you should figure that out. Due to chronic (and perhaps escalating) consumption over the years, you've also probably become so desensitized to caffeine that it's not injecting you with you nearly as much pep as it used to. So give it up for a while, reintroduce it, and compare your experiences.

Two words of caution here. First, on the Energy Reset, it may take you longer than 30 days to see results. It's not because of the fat adaption process; that starts in just a few days, and most Whole30ers report feeling steady energy throughout the day by their third week into the program. Withdrawing from caffeine, however, can disrupt your energy levels and sleep for many weeks*, depending on the severity of your habit. If you design your reset for 30 days but find you still aren't where you want to be energy-wise, consider extending your reset by 15 to 30 days to see if you can't continue to recover energy levels naturally.

Second, your energy will get worse before it gets better. During the in-between stages—when you're no longer giving your body sugar all the time, but aren't very good at using fat as fuel—you'll likely feel lethargic, cranky, and foggy. This usually improves by the second week of the program, but if you don't know it's coming, it may chip away at your commitment to the reset. Get lots of sleep, go easy in the gym or at your sport, and make sure you're eating enough to support your activity levels—this, too, shall pass.

DON'T BE CARB-PHOBIC

This is not a low-carb plan by design. You'll likely be eating fewer carbohydrates as a result of your food choices, but you'll still be eating them, especially if you're active or enjoy high-intensity exercise. Don't be afraid of potatoes, winter squashes, beets, taro, yuca or cassava, plantains, and any other form of fresh fruit! (Yes, you've been warned on other diets that bananas and potatoes are too sugary to be healthy, but here, in the context of only eating real food and training your body to be better at managing energy, that's just silly.) Mix them in with the leafy greens and other nutrient-dense veggies to create a healthy balance of carbohydrates in your daily diet. In fact, if your energy is improving, then suddenly takes a turn for the worse, it's probably because you've been undereating carbohydrates. Try including at least a fist-size portion of carb-dense vegetables and/or fruit with every meal for a few days, and see if things improve.

* When I gave up caffeine for good in 2010, it took me just two weeks to regain my energy, but about six weeks for my sleep to improve. However, if I can write four books and survive a newborn baby without caffeine, you can manage for 30 days—#toughlove.

VEGAN RESET

On this reset, you'll be completely eliminating the following foods and beverages (in addition to no animal products):

- Gluten-containing grains
- Peanuts
- Alcohol
- Added sugar
- Artificial sweeteners
- Sweets/treats/baked goods

If you're a staunch vegan, it's impossible to do the Whole30 as written, as the program eliminates nearly all your plant-based protein sources. Still, it's entirely possible for you to eliminate some of the most commonly problematic foods (specifically, gluten-containing grains and peanuts) to see how they are impacting you. In addition, to properly reset your hormones and emotional attachments to certain foods, you'll want to adopt a Whole30-ish program without alcohol, added sugar, or vegan "treats."

Soy is one of the most commonly allergenic foods, but also a staple in a vegan diet. It would be very hard to eliminate all forms of soy during your reset, so to keep your soy consumption as healthy as possible, choose organic and/or fermented forms (like organic tofu, tempeh, or natto) and unprocessed forms like edamame over processed soy products like veggie burgers.

Beans are high-FODMAP foods, which commonly produce digestive distress. If you know beans don't work well for you, it may be wise to leave them out of your reset, reintroducing them one group at a time to see how you fare. (Note that products made from soy protein, like tempeh or tofu, don't fall into this category, but the soybean itself does, so if this is your context, you may want eliminate edamame and avoid all forms of soy milk.)

You should also consider prolonged soaking, extended cooking, rinsing, sprouting, and/or fermenting your gluten-free grains, beans, nuts, and seeds. This time-honored practice reduces their anti-nutrient content (compounds that reduce the absorption of nutrients), releasing beneficial vitamins and minerals and making them more bioavailable.

Pseudo-cereals tend to be less problematic in the gut than actual grain-based protein sources, especially those that contain gluten (like seitan), and some are "complete proteins," containing all of the essential amino acids. Try supplementing your non-gluten grains and legumes with quinoa, spelt, Kamut, teff, amaranth, and sorghum as part of a more varied diet.

Don't attempt to eat your body weight in grams of protein as a vegan, as many plant-based sources (like beans) actually contain far more carbohydrates than protein. You'll already be getting carbohydrates from vegetables and fruit, so deliberately upping your protein can inadvertently send your total carbs skyrocketing, potentially creating hormonal imbalances and blood sugar regulation issues. One way to mitigate this is to include lots of healthy fats in your diet (from coconut products, avocado, olives and olive oil, nuts, and seeds), which serves two purposes. First, high-fat diets have been shown to be muscle-sparing—good for those eating less protein. Second, eating more fat will help keep your body good at using fat as fuel, reducing your cravings for sugar when you need energy.

As part of your reset, you'll get all your protein from real food sources, skipping plant-based protein powders. These meal replacements or supplements don't provide much protein per serving, usually include less-healthy fillers, and are always sweetened with some form of sugar or stevia.

NOT QUITE VEGAN?

If you avoid most animal protein but are comfortable eating eggs and seafood, I'd strongly encourage you to do the Whole30 over a vegan reset. The inclusion of some naturally raised animal products in your reset diet will make you healthier, and doing the Whole30 will help you evaluate the impact the plant-based protein sources you've been eating are actually having on you. It may get a bit tedious to eat nothing but eggs and seafood as your protein sources for 30 days, but the end result—a complete reset, and newfound awareness of how foods like soy or seitan are impacting your health—is worth it. Check out the hundreds of delicious egg- and seafood-based recipes on the @whole30recipes Instagram feed to stave off food boredom.

BASIC RESET

On this reset, you'll be completely eliminating the following foods and beverages:

- Gluten-containing grains
- Dairy
- Alcohol

LIMIT

- Added sugar
- Artificial sweeteners
- Processed foods

The Basic Reset looks a little different than the others. You'll note there's less to exclude and more gray area. (What does "limiting processed foods" mean to you? How much sugar is too much?)

This plan is designed for those who are hungry for a change but don't have the emotional capacity to "go big." The Basic Reset might appeal to you if the idea of giving up *all* the foods outlined in other resets is just too daunting; you're not emotionally prepared to make huge, all-in changes; or you strongly prefer moderation to abstaining. Before you celebrate, however (yay, dark chocolate could still be on the table!), it's time for some more tough love.

First, this plan requires even more self-awareness and self-discipline than the others. (Translation: Your willpower bank had better be full.) Since there are fewer black-and-white rules, you'll have to rely on your own best judgment to make decisions about what foods are okay during your reset. Is dark chocolate really okay if you're trying to change your relationship with sugar? Is a fast-food burger and fries (even if you hold the bun) an appropriate part of this process? Is that alternative-flour muffin really going to help you break your comfort food habits?

You know my take on all of these.

In the moment, using your best judgment (especially if you're coming from a place where you're not always entirely in control of your food) is going to be really challenging. It would be way easier to simply follow one of the black-and-white plans, and you'd expend far less willpower that way, too. Just sayin'.

In addition, this plan isn't likely to work as well as any of the others, because it's not making the kind of serious change that a true reset demands. It has a pretty good chance of helping you feel at least somewhat better, giving you the self-confidence boost, energy, and motivation you need to keep you moving toward better health and improved habits. But it's not going to deliver the same magic that a stronger protocol will, which means you may not emerge on the other side feeling as different as you'd hoped.

Finally, one last piece of tough love (heavy on the love): To find food freedom, you must be prepared to follow at least the Basic Reset: eliminating all forms of gluten, dairy, and alcohol; keeping all foods and beverages minimally processed; and steering clear of added sugar or artificial sweeteners. This is the *bare minimum* of any effective reset, and should only be used when you truly don't have the capacity to change your diet any more dramatically.

If you're unwilling to completely eliminate even this stuff, don't bother continuing.

If you don't totally eliminate at least these items, it's going to be impossible to effect a lasting change. Which means you'll spend the next 30 days giving up foods you really like, learning nothing from the process, and seeing little to no transformation as a result.

That last sentence would make a terrible ad campaign.

So do what you need to do to mentally and physically prepare yourself and your environment for at least the elimination of gluten, dairy, alcohol, and processed foods for the next month or two, because this is your ticket to lasting food freedom—and you're here because you're ready to make some real changes this time, changes that stick.

DO HARD THINGS

here is another benefit of taking on any reset, beyond physiological changes or health improvements. That benefit comes from committing to something you know will be really challenging, and finishing what you started. Your connection to food is highly emotional, which is part of why diet is one of the hardest habits to change. If you're scared to try even the Basic Reset, that's okay! Giving up the foods you've been relying on for comfort, love, and reward is a scary proposition. But find the motivation you need to commit, take it on, and SEE IT THROUGH, because the self-confidence this experience brings will spill over into every other area of your life. Prove to yourself that you can do hard things, and there's nothing that won't be impacted in a positive way.

Tips for a Successful Reset

Whatever your approach, there are things you should do along the way to ensure a successful reset—and one thing that could sabotage your efforts, if you're not aware of it.

First, maintain awareness throughout the entire reset process, and take good notes. A journal can be helpful in identifying and documenting changes in your sleep, energy levels, mood, digestion, athletic performance, or medical symptoms. Note anything that feels significant, even if it's small, to see if you can spot a pattern the next time you eat that same food or drink that same beverage. Rate subjective things like energy or joint pain on a scale of 1 to 10, use a wearable fitness device to track things like sleep and steps taken, and make note of fitness metrics before, during, and after the experiment. If you have a medical condition like high cholesterol or diabetes, you may want to have your doctor run some baseline tests before your reset, and compare them to measurements taken at the end of your program. (And that first visit is a great opportunity to run your reset plan by your doctor.)

Before-and-after photos can also be incredibly helpful, as physical changes can happen so slowly that you may not notice them from day to day. Taking pictures of skin conditions (acne, eczema, or psoriasis), joint swelling (like your knuckles), or full-body photos to compare body composition or stomach bloating are encouraged before, during, and after your reset. These photos can also provide you with continued motivation, as you see small improvements happening throughout the process.

Second, remember that planning and preparation are the key to any successful reset. The more robust your plan for grocery shopping, meals, social gatherings, travel delays, and stressful times, the more successful you'll be in sticking to the plan. Here are some general tips that apply to any reset:

CHOOSE YOUR START DATE. Look at the calendar and find a reasonable time to complete the reset, taking into account 10 days at the end for reintroduction. Ideally, you will start ASAP. Birthday parties, business dinners, and family gatherings aren't an excuse to put it off—you'll have to figure out how to eat this way in all kinds of "normal" life situations, so write these into your plan for the month and plunge in. A once-in-a-lifetime trip to Italy, your wedding week, or the month your new baby is due, though, are legitimate excuses to delay taking on this challenge. Still, find the right time as soon as you can, before your momentum stalls.

REMOVE ANY AND ALL ELIMINATION FOODS FROM YOUR HOME (or condense your family's treats into one cabinet or refrigerator drawer so you're not moving the cookies every time you need a can of coconut milk). This is important. You'll think you won't need to do this, because you've read this book, and are feeling strong and motivated. Do it anyway. Future You will thank you for it.

PLAN YOUR MEALS AS FAR AHEAD AS IS COMFORTABLE. Make sure you always have compliant emergency food on hand for those stuck-at-the-airport/long-business-meeting/soccer-game-went-into-overtime moments. (Visit whole30.com/whole30-approved for my favorite healthy convenience foods.) Figure out when you'll have time to meal prep and batch cook, and how often it's reasonable for you to grocery shop.

GO SHOPPING! Stock up on reset staples you may not have on hand (like healthy cooking oils or spices), and buy what you'll need to get you started on your meal plan.

ANTICIPATE POTENTIALLY CHALLENGING SITUATIONS. Then, make a plan for how you'll handle them, so you feel comfortable sticking to your reset at those birthday parties, business dinners, and family gatherings. (Refer to page 17 in *The Whole30*; even if you're not doing our program, our preparatory tips will still be super helpful.)

SEEK SOCIAL SUPPORT AND ACCOUNTABILITY. This is critical whether you choose to do the Whole30 or create your own reset. Habit research shows that support from others can help you maintain your motivation, impact your actions and intentions by modeling the desired behavior (which is why I recommend you join a like-minded online forum or social media community during your reset), and reduce stress by providing an environment for healthy interpersonal connection, which helps you better manage negative emotions and stay on track.

FIND YOUR TRIBE

If you do the Whole30, you can join our free online forum and participate in our social media communities (see page 236). If you're creating your own reset, search for groups (vegan, vegetarian, Paleo, gluten-free, AIP, etc.) who will help you support your plan. You can also use the strategies I outline in chapter 12 for talking to family, friends, and co-workers about your new health initiative to gain in-person support.

One more thing: Don't let your reset turn you into a hermit. You're eating healthy, not battling an infectious disease. There is no reason you can't continue to socialize, dine out, attend parties and events, and travel during your reset. It just requires a bit more planning and preparation, and a mind-shift away from thinking these special occasions are about the food. They're not. They're about the people you're with, the laughter you'll share, the traditions you'll create, and the stress-moderating effect of in-person social interaction. So research the menu, pack your emergency food, bring your own side dish, be ready with your order of seltzer water with lime, and get out there during your reset. (For tips and tricks on dining out and travel during your reset, visit whole30.com/pdf-downloads.)

Now, a final word of caution: Nothing sabotages your reset faster than focusing only on the technicalities while ignoring the spirit and intention of your program. Here's an example: You're doing a vegan reset and have eliminated your beloved nondairy ice cream and baked goods, but you're still craving something sweet after dinner every night. Then you discover sliced bananas covered in melted coconut butter and cacao nibs (or fried plantain chips, or Cherry Pie flavored fruit-and-nut bars), and that becomes your after-dinner "dessert."

Is that technically compliant? Yes. Is it in the spirit of a reset, designed to change your habits and your emotional relationship with food (and in this case, dessert)? Decidedly not.

It's your program. You have to own it.

Remember that your reset isn't just about following the technicality of the rules. You really have to ask yourself the tough questions: Is using a certain substitute food to satisfy a craving really what you want for your reset? Do you still feel in control when you eat that food? Are you impulsively reaching for something sweet, fatty, salty, or crunchy because you're feeling anxious, lonely, or bored? Are you changing your bad habits here, or just continuing them with less-bad foods? If you didn't reach for this food to satisfy this craving or emotion, what else could you do to treat or comfort yourself?

There are ways to finish the reset without actually resetting a thing— and ways to complete the program that will change your life in a dramatic and permanent fashion. The devil is in the details, and the clearer you are about your goals and the more aware you can be throughout the process, the more success you will have with your program.

And with that . . . it's time to reset! You've totally got this, but just in case you get stuck, come on over to the Whole30 community for support; we'll help you out, even if your reset looks a little different. (I'd say "See you in 30 days," but we both know you're so excited about this whole "food freedom" thing that you're already turning the page.)

CHAPTER 5

THE RESET (REINTRODUCTION)

Now that your reset is done, it's time to eat All the Things! You've been so good, surely you deserve a reward . . . right? You know better by now. That's something you used to do with those old quick-fix weight-loss plans, but it isn't at all the right mind-set for a reset. Still, it may be hard to shake the idea that your "diet" is "over" and you can return to old favorite foods and habits; an idea that will compromise your motivation to follow a proper reintroduction. But remember, reintroduction is mission-critical to your Food Freedom plan. To reduce the chance that you'll blow this off, you need to shift your mind-set from "diet" to "reset," so let's take a page straight out of habit research.

A 2010 study in the *Journal of Abnormal Psychology* examined craving levels among flight attendants during a short flight (3 to 5½ hours long) and a long flight (8 to 13 hours long). All flight attendants recruited for the study were smokers. You'd assume that cravings would be much worse during the long flight, as the flight attendants knew they couldn't smoke again for quite some time. What the study actually found, however, was that cravings weren't tied to flight duration, but to the *time remaining* in the flight, when the brain perceived a reward in sight. In fact, craving levels at the three-hour mark of the short flight were actually much higher than the three-hour mark of the long flight. Why? Because the short flight was about to land, and the attendants knew a cigarette (reward) was on the horizon.

What do jonesing flight attendants have to do with your reset?

A large body of evidence shows that cravings are largely determined by environmental cues and expectations. Thinking about your reset "ending" is the same as knowing your plane is about to land; your brain believes that a reward is imminent. To combat this, simply think about your reset as moving in phases, with no definite beginning and end. Yes, the elimination portion was 30 days, and today it's Day 31 . . . but it's not *over*; you're simply moving into the reintroduction phase. After which you'll move into the Food Freedom phase. And after that, the oops-I'm-back-to-drinking-wine-after-work-every-day phase (because I told you this would happen), which brings you right back to the reset phase.

See? It's not over—you're just ready to start the next chapter, where you'll get to reintroduce some of the delicious foods you've been missing, while still paying careful attention to the experience and remaining fully in control. That sounds way healthier than rebounding with a sugar-fat-salt fiesta, doesn't it?

WE'RE NOT DIETING

To reinforce this point, continue to bring yourself back to this idea every time you get stuck in a diet mind-set. *This* is not *that*. You're not dieting. You're not deprived. You're not desperately chasing quick weight loss. You are conscientiously resetting your health, habits, and relationship with food; creating the perfect, balanced, sustainable diet; and taking control of the food you are eating—even the "less healthy" stuff. Write it down if you have to: "I am not dieting." You've never done this kind of program before, so you'll have to work hard to change the way you think about it. It's understandable if that takes time—just keep reminding yourself, and eventually, it will stick.

On the opposite end of the spectrum, you may be feeling guilty or anxious about the thought of reintroducing the foods you've been missing. You'll bring bread, wine, or chocolate back in because you've missed it so much and want to know how it's going to impact you, but then you won't allow yourself to enjoy the experience because you feel so darn *guilty* about it.

This is not food freedom.

Remember, you didn't eliminate your reset foods because they were bad or unhealthy, you eliminated them to see how they worked for you. The point isn't to give them up forever; it's to evaluate the impact they have on your body and brain, and then decide what role *you* want them to play in your new, healthy lifestyle.

There is no guilt in this. It's just part of the process. Let's go back to the pet analogy:

Say you have a dog. Every day, you wake up and your nose is a little itchy, your eyes are a little red, and your throat is scratchy. You love your dog, but you recognize that you don't feel well, and you'd like to feel better. You start to wonder if your dog is the culprit. So in an effort to figure out your sensitivities, you send your dog to your mom's house for a month.

You really miss your dog, so when the month is up, you want to see whether you can bring him back into the house without firing up your allergies. So you go pick him up and bring him home.

Do you feel guilty about bringing your dog back? Of course not! In fact, you're psyched to see him, crossing your fingers that you can have him around without getting stuffy again. And yay! After some trial and error, you discovered you can. So you happily invite him back home to stay, because you love your dog and you've figured out that as long as he's not sleeping on your bed and gets bathed once a week, you can have your dog and still maintain a mostly allergy-free existence.

This is winning.

In the elimination/reintroduction scenario, your dog = bread. (Or wine, or cheese . . .)

You've missed it. You love it. You're still not sure if it's going to work for you, but *that's why you reintroduce.* Don't feel guilty about it. Embrace it. Enjoy it. Savor the return of the delicious, special foods you've been missing, and then figure out whether you want to include those foods in your new life in some capacity.

Reintroduction is a necessary step toward food freedom. So is losing the idea that foods are universally "good" or "bad." Remember, even if these foods don't work for you, that still doesn't make them unhealthy, just *less healthy for you.*

Reintroduction Reinforcement

Reintroduction should take between 10 and 30 days and is not to be rushed! Foods must be reintroduced one at a time, while maintaining the reset diet. Think of it like a scientific experiment, where you're looking to systematically evaluate just one factor at a time to see how it impacts you. If, on Day 31, you run right out and eat pizza, ice cream, and beer, how will you know if the gluten in the pizza crust or the milk in the mint chocolate chip made your face break out? Was it the beer or the cheese that made your belly bloat? Did the sugar, the processed carbs, or the alcohol tank your energy?

At the risk of sounding like a broken record, remember that the reintroduction phase is just as crucial to complete as outlined as the elimination. Without reintroducing the foods and drinks you've cut out carefully and systematically, one at a time, you'll never know how individual foods are affecting your energy, sleep, mood, cravings, digestion, symptoms, or medical condition. You'll miss the opportunity to compare how you look and feel *without* these foods to how you look and feel when you consume them. And you won't have the critical information you need to create the perfect diet for you.

Without a proper elimination and reintroduction, there is no food freedom.

Let's return to the pet analogy. Again, you have five pets (a dog, two cats, the rabbit, and a bird), and again, you're feeling stuffy, wheezy, and itchy. In an effort to diagnose the cause of your symptoms, you send all your pets to your mom's, and you don't go visit them at all—no contact except for Facetime. (They love Facetime.) When the month is over, you feel amazing—allergy symptoms are totally gone! To celebrate, you have your mom bring all your pets back home to you, and you have a reunion group-snuggle with them all at once. The next morning, you wake up, and all your allergy symptoms are back with a vengeance.

So now you know that your animals are definitely contributing to your allergies. But do you know *which* animals may be the culprit? Nope. Are you just as physically miserable as the day you gave them away? Yes—perhaps more so, because now you know how good you could be feeling. Have you put yourself and your pets through a month of hardship and learned virtually nothing from the process? Yes, that's exactly what you've done.

It might feel hard, but substitute bread, wine, cheese, cookies, and peanut butter for the animals. Now imagine trying to figure out which of these commonly problematic foods has been negatively impacting your energy, sleep, cravings, bloating, acne, allergies, asthma, migraines, joint pain, hives, or depression when you reintroduce them all into your diet *at the same time*.

You can't.

In summary, you have to eliminate *and* reintroduce carefully and systematically. It's the fastest and easiest way to know how the foods you've been eating are impacting you. In fact, most medical doctors agree that a structured elimination diet is the most effective way to identify food sensitivities—more so than lab tests in many cases. And it's the reintroduction phase that tells you which foods are actually worth it, and which make you feel so poorly, you're happy to live without them.

Reintroduction Guidelines

The Whole30 outlined two different sample reintroduction schedules, and I welcome you to borrow them if you want some guidance. However, you don't have to follow a set schedule or specific reintroduction food order. The key is reintroducing just one variable at a time and leaving enough space (generally two to three days) between reintroduction food groups to allow any side effects to present themselves and subside.

On the designated reintroduction day, you'll want to reintroduce enough of that food group to really test the effects. If you just have one sip of milk on dairy day, you may not notice anything, which may lead you to believe that milk is totally fine. While that approach may sound appealing ("I reintroduced and everything was okay!"), you want to "go big" here, too, and really subject your body and brain to the potential negative effects of these previously eliminated foods. Reintroduce several items from that food group throughout the course of your reintroduction day. That means on dairy day, you'll put cream in your coffee, drink milk with breakfast, eat a yogurt with lunch, and liberally sprinkle cheese on your dinner salad.

The exception here is alcohol. Let's not get drunk before noon, m'kay? Try no more than two glasses of your favorite beverage with dinner—trust me, that will be enough to evaluate the impact.

Ideally, you're reintroducing foods in order of *least* likely to be problematic to *most* likely to be problematic, but this is hard if you're not sure which foods are going to negatively impact you. A rule of thumb: Added sugar, gluten-free alcohol (like wine), legumes, and non-gluten grains can be reintroduced toward the beginning, but save dairy and gluten for the very last phases. (Again, you can use the sample reintroduction scheduled outlined in *The Whole30* to guide you here, even if you've designed your own reset.)

Reintroducing sugar is hard, as it almost always comes tied in with other food groups (like gluten or dairy). If you want to see what reintroducing sugar alone feels like, add sweetener to your morning coffee, drizzle honey over your sweet potato at lunch, have a sweet tea in the afternoon, and enjoy some poached peaches with maple syrup after dinner. Then, when you reintroduce other food groups that also contain sugar (like flavored yogurt or a muffin), you'll be able to compare the effects of eating *just* sugar with eating sugar plus that other food group.

It's tough to come up with a comprehensive list of everything that could happen when you reintroduce these potentially less-healthy foods, because various components of different foods interact with every single person in a unique fashion. You're looking for any noticeable changes—a reversal of improvement, a return to not-so-awesome, a decline in performance, or a resurgence of symptoms.

Sometimes it's obvious; if you suddenly look three months pregnant, your skin breaks out, your sweet tooth acts up, or your joints swell or hurt again, that's a pretty clear indicator that the reintroduced item isn't making you healthier. Whole30 alumna Kelsey discovered this for herself when she reintroduced dairy in the form of a milkshake. Within 20 minutes, she was doubled over in stomach pain, and she remained bloated and gassy for a few days. Kelsey was shocked at the impact of dairy on her system, saying, "I knew gluten upset me, and I'd had gall bladder issues in the past, but I didn't ever suspect that dairy would be so problematic. Now I know, so I will just stay away from it unless it's *really* worth it."

However, keep an eye out for the subtleties, too. Maybe it's a little tougher to wake up in the morning, your focus at work at 2 p.m. isn't quite as sharp, your mood takes a sharp turn for the bummed, or you find yourself prowling through the pantry more frequently.

REINTRODUCTION IDEAS

You may be finding it hard to reintroduce just that one food group on any given day, when most of the stuff you want to eat includes more than one potentially problematic ingredient. Rule of thumb: Keep reintroduction foods minimally processed and generally low in added sugar, so you can evaluate just one factor at a time. Here are some examples:

NON-GLUTEN GRAINS: corn on the cob, homemade popcorn with ghee or clarified butter, 100% corn tortillas, gluten-free oatmeal, white or brown rice, a side of quinoa

DAIRY: heavy cream or full-fat milk, butter, plain yogurt or kefir, cheese, cottage cheese, cream cheese, whey protein powder

GLUTEN-CONTAINING GRAINS: whole-grain bread, wraps, or tortillas; pasta or couscous; crackers; low-sugar whole-grain cereals

GLUTEN-CONTAINING ALCOHOL: beer

GLUTEN-FREE ALCOHOL: gluten-free beer or cider, wine, and unflavored vodka, tequila, gin, rum, or any distilled (unflavored) spirits.*

*Distilled spirits, even those made from wheat, rye, or barley, are generally considered gluten-free. Anecdotally, however, many gluten-sensitive individuals stay away from rye, whiskey, Scotch, bourbon, and vodkas made from wheat. While the University of Chicago Celiac Disease Center says the distillation process makes these liquors safe, use your own judgment.

PAY ATTENTION

Here is a list of things you could evaluate during the reintroduction phase, to determine if a particular food is having a negative impact on you:

- Digestion
- Energy
- Sleep
- Cravings
- Mood/happiness
- Attention span/focus
- Self-confidence
- Skin

- Allergies
- Breathing (asthma, congestion)
- Headaches/migraines
- Athletic performance or recovery
- Pain
- Inflammation
- Medical symptoms

SAMPLE REINTRODUCTION SCHEDULE
(BASED ON THE CRAVING-BUSTER RESET)

DAYS 1–30: Elimination

DAY 31: Reintroduce nuts and seeds, all by themselves (almond butter on your apple with breakfast, a handful of macadamias with lunch, and toasted almonds on your dinner salad)

DAYS 32–33: Back to the strict elimination diet

DAY 34: Reintroduce non-gluten grains all by themselves (gluten-free oatmeal for breakfast, quinoa mixed into your lunch salad, and 100% corn tortillas instead of lettuce wraps for dinner)

DAYS 35–36: Back to the strict elimination diet

DAY 37: Reintroduce dairy, all by itself (heavy cream in your coffee, cheddar cheese in your breakfast omelet, plain Greek yogurt with lunch, and feta over your zucchini noodles at dinner)

DAYS 38–39: Back to the strict elimination diet

DAY 40: Reintroduce gluten-containing grains, all by themselves (whole wheat flakes with unsweetened almond milk for breakfast, a sandwich for lunch, and whole wheat pasta with dinner)

DAYS 41–42: Back to the strict elimination diet

DAY 43: Reintroduce alcohol, all by itself (two glasses of beer, wine, potato vodka, or tequila)

DAY 44–45: Back to the strict elimination diet

DAY 46: Reintroduce added sugars, including dried fruit, all by themselves (sugar in your coffee, a dried-fruit-and-nut bar with lunch, brown sugar and ghee over your sweet potato at dinner)

DAY 47–48: Back to the strict elimination diet

DAY 49: Reintroduce baked goods, sweets, and treats, ideally gluten- and dairy-free (a gluten-free muffin with breakfast, a handful of date-and-coconut balls with lunch, and some dark chocolate with your tea after dinner)

And while Days 46 and 49 sound like the *best days ever*, eating this much sugar, baked goods, and sweets in a short period of time is seriously likely to be problematic. UNDERSTATEMENT. Pay really close attention here; your Sugar Dragon will likely awaken with a vengeance, and may require several additional days of reset to calm.

Repeat this process based on the foods you've eliminated during your specific reset until everything has been reintroduced and carefully evaluated. You can break this schedule down as detailed as you like, too—reintroduction could easily stretch out for another full 30 days or longer. If you want to evaluate cheese separately from other forms of dairy, make that two different sessions. If you miss corn a ton, but those other gluten-grains not so much, do a corn-only day (try corn tortillas with your breakfast eggs, baked tortilla chips and salsa with lunch, and corn on the cob with dinner), waiting a few days before testing out other non-gluten grains.

Finally, remember that the impact of these potentially less-healthy foods adds up. If at any point you feel like you haven't adequately recovered from the effects of the reintroduced foods, give yourself a few more days between food groups. Allow the side effects to settle before adding anything else, as the point is to bring the eliminated foods back into a "clean" environment so you can properly evaluate their impact.

NOT MISSING IT?

I f you're not missing a particular food that you suspect is making you less healthy, don't bother reintroducing it. Waffles weren't your thing? Skip them on Day 46! Don't care about testing how wine impacts you because you feel so good without it? Skip the alcohol reintroduction for now. Remember, reintroduction is a lifelong process, so you can always leave something out of this structured timeline, and just pay attention later if it comes across your field of vision and you decide you want to test the waters.

During your reintroduction process, you'll be bombarded with lots of information coming at you all at once. The changes to your energy, sleep, mood, cravings, digestion, skin, joints, athletic performance, recovery, and medical symptoms may be numerous and overlapping. It may be difficult to remember exactly how individual meals or specific foods impacted you physically, psychologically, and emotionally during this time period if you aren't writing at least some of it down.

You probably won't want to do this. It sounds like even more effort, when you've already been working so hard. You'll think it feels like overkill. This is just your brain trying to convince you not to remember, because boy, will it want you to bring some of these foods back into your life, regardless of the consequences.

Which is exactly why you should listen to me, and not the toddler inside your head screaming for a cookie.

Keep a reintroduction journal either on paper, in your computer, or in the Notes app on your smartphone. It can be as simple or as detailed as you'd like to make it, although the more detail you add, the better prepared you'll be to make good choices for yourself going forward. Create a new entry for each day, and track how things go after each reintroduced item. Evaluate the same things that improved on your Non-Scale Victory checklist (page 33) and write a summary of your thoughts and experiences at the end of each day. A sample reintroduction journal day might look like this:

7 A.M. Added sugar to my coffee. It tasted good, but I'm used to drinking it black now. Won't do this again.

8 A.M. Veggie frittata and side of berries with breakfast. Topped my berries at breakfast with some maple syrup. Way too sweet. Fruit does not need sugar.

10 A.M. Feeling good, no cravings.

11:30 A.M. Giant protein salad for lunch + honey in my tea. It was good. The end.

2 P.M. Snack: That Banana Bread dried-fruit-and-nut bar was delicious. Like candy. So happy. I ate two. Oops.

3 P.M. My head is on my desk. This hasn't happened in a month. Shoot.

4 P.M. I want another dried-fruit-and-nut bar. Or that leftover muffin on the counter. Or the candy in my co-worker's jar. Anything. I'll take anything. MUST RESIST.

6 P.M. Stuffed peppers with pesto for dinner, skipping the brown sugar on my roasted butternut squash. I just don't want it.

9 P.M. I'm back to prowling the pantry looking for something sweet. Damn you, sugar! Back to my reset for a few days, until my Sugar Dragon calms down.

END OF DAY THOUGHTS: When I add sugar to meals, it doesn't seem to be a big deal. When I eat it by itself (snack or dessert), my cravings came back with a vengeance, and I felt out of control again. I'm going to be really careful with stand-alone treats and desserts going forward.

Ultimately, when you've reintroduced every food and drink you've been missing, have paid close attention to what changes (for better or worse) when you eat them, and have a good understanding of how these items impact your health, habits, and relationship with food . . . you're done with your reset! So how did it go?

Evaluating Your Reset

By the time your reset is over, you should feel like a brand-new person. (Yes, I set the standard that high, mostly because that's how nearly all Whole30ers report feeling by Day 31.) Your energy should be rocking, your sleep improved, your digestion better, and your tummy flatter. Your skin will be glowing, and your aches and pains will have diminished. That annoying *thing* that used to happen? It isn't happening anymore. And everyone wants to know, "What have you been doing?" You're happier, more self-confident, and your cravings are dramatically reduced. In fact, you don't even *want* most of the foods you couldn't wait to devour when your reset was over, because you just feel so good.

Oh, and your pants may be looser, too, which wasn't the point, but is still pretty sweet.

You've also learned an incredible amount in a very short time about how the foods you've been eating have been affecting you. You can draw clear lines between eating X food and seeing Y effect on your body, energy, or mood. Your awareness and self-control are at an all-time high, built on a solid foundation of changed tastes, improved blood sugar regulation, more evenly balanced hormones, a healthier digestive tract, and a calmer immune system. In other words, you've successfully pushed the reset button on your health, habits, and relationship with food.

This *is* how you feel, right?

If the answer is yes, high five! You've successfully taken the first step toward lifelong food freedom. But if you're not feeling this way, that's okay, too. Not even the Whole30 works this well for everyone who tries it, and if you've designed your own plan, I did mention that you may need some tweaks along the way (or a few attempts) before you found yourself fully "reset."

But before you throw in the towel and accept the idea that your reset "just didn't work," let's troubleshoot the most common scenarios.

YOU DIDN'T GO "BIG" ENOUGH. If you didn't do the full Whole30 or one of the more comprehensive elimination plans, there's a good chance you still have things in your diet that are negatively impacting you; keeping your cravings alive, energy in flux, digestion disrupted, and immune system active. *Solution:* Go bigger! Do the Whole30 by the book or work with a functional medicine doctor (page 235) to design an elimination plan specifically for you.

ANOTHER PUSH FOR WHOLE30

I f your self-designed reset wasn't everything you hoped it would be, I'll encourage you *one more time* to try the Whole30. The plan's structure, incredible social support, and extensive resources may be just what you need to push you over the edge from feeling so-so about your reset to feeling like your entire life just changed. Oh, and do it now. Yes, right now. Don't wait, don't give yourself a month "off," and don't tell yourself you'll start after this holiday or that special event. Do it *now*, while you're still in "healthy eating" mode, and build on the improvements you *did* see during your self-designed reset. By Day 31 of your Whole30, I'd be shocked if you didn't reread the first few paragraphs of this section and say, "Well, NOW I understand what she was talking about!"

YOU DIDN'T DO IT RIGHT. Yeah, I said it, because this process demands some serious self-analysis. Did you *really* stick to your reset 100%? Did you truly embrace the spirit and intention of the program, not just the technicalities? (Translation: Did you just complete 30 days full of egg-and-banana "pancakes"; late-night dried fruit with coconut butter snacks; and bacon-wrapped, cashew butter–stuffed dates? I know that last thing sounds amazing, but stay focused here.) Did you really focus on improving your health, or were you so stuck on weight loss that you took your reset to an unhealthy place, cutting calories, restricting fruit, or deliberately eating low-fat? *Solution:* Do it again. Do it right. The end.

THIRTY DAYS WASN'T LONG ENOUGH. While radical health improvements can take place in just 30 days, when you put it into context, decades of less-than-healthy behavior often can't compete with just one month of new action. Resetting your metabolism takes time, especially if you've been eating a Standard American Diet (SAD) for years. And fixing an unhealthy psychological relationship with food—plus the cravings, habits, and emotional ties that go along with one—is often the toughest battle to win. If you're feeling better but were hoping for more improvements (especially if you feel like your cravings aren't yet under control), extending your plan a bit longer may help. *Solution:* Return to your reset for another 15 to 30 days, and see if that brings you the "magic" you seek.

YOU'RE PAYING ATTENTION TO THE WRONG THINGS. You really, really wanted to lose weight, but you didn't lose weight, or you didn't lose as much as you had hoped. So you deem the reset a failure, because the number on the scale didn't budge. *Solution:* This fix has more to do with gaining perspective and less to do with the need for a new or longer reset. I'm also betting you chose not to journal your experience along the way, which is why you're not able to really see and recognize all the improvements you've made. Reevaluate what *else* happened during your reset. Go back to the Non-Scale Victory Checklist (remember that, from page 33?) and mark off everything that got better during the program, no matter how small. Ask yourself, Why am I still giving my scale this much power? Isn't it finally time to give that up? (It is. You'll thank me.)

DIET ISN'T YOUR BIGGEST ISSUE. If you're coming from a SAD (even a "healthy" one, focused on whole grains and low-fat everything), I'd be shocked if the Whole30 or one of the bigger resets proposed here didn't dramatically improve how you look, feel, and live. But if you can honestly say you went pretty big, followed it 100%, and still aren't checking many things off your #NSV sheet, then it's time to look at other factors. *Solution:* Find a functional medicine practitioner to help you figure out why you're still not feeling well, but maintain your healthy reset diet, because asking if you've eliminated gluten, dairy, and processed foods will be the first thing a good practitioner will do. Once you've implemented your doctor's treatment plan, you can return to this book knowing you've got all the factors in place to properly reset and move forward.

Building a Life of Food Freedom

So now you've got a complete reset plan: how to eliminate, how to reintroduce, what to pay attention to along the way, and how to correct if you find your chosen method of reset wasn't as effective as you'd hoped. Congratulations! Your reset is over!

Um, now what?

First, I'll tell you what's *not* next: a sharp drop into an abyss of "That was great and I feel amazing but I'm totally lost on what to do next." That's what happened with all your *other* diets, but as you've been reminding yourself all along, *this* is not *that*.

Now I'm going to give you a detailed road map for taking what you've learned during your reset and turning those lessons into a balanced diet that's perfect for you. I'll tell you how to sustain, even in times of stress, the new, healthy habits you created during your reset. I'll teach you how to talk to family and friends about your new lifestyle, which common situations are most likely to throw you off your healthy-eating game, how to recover when you slide back into old habits, and how to maintain the food freedom you've found for the rest of your life.

Translation: This time, you have a plan.

Feel better? Good. Now take a moment to be proud of your hard work and achievements, and bask in the glory of feeling totally in control of the food you're eating for the first time in a long while.

And when you're done with *that* . . . take a deep breath, because there's still work to be done.

ENJOYING YOUR FOOD FREEDOM

CHAPTER 6

FOOD FREEDOM, DEFINED

Your reset is over and you've successfully reintroduced; now you're ready to make your own decisions out there in the real world. The Whole30 calls this "riding your own bike," because once your reset training wheels come off and you're setting your own guidelines, it's equal parts exhilarating and terrifying.

You may be excited to jump straight into your new, healthy diet and apply what you learned during your reset. If that's the case, excellent! This section features a great plan to keep you on track and in control while reincorporating the "less-healthy-but-still-worth-it" foods you've missed.

More likely, you're nervous about bringing stuff back in. You feel so good right now, and you're afraid that without the structure of the reintroduction to keep you in check, that first hit of sugar, processed carbs, wine, or cheese will send you rebounding straight back into your old habits. You may be so scared that you want to stay on the reset 24/7/365—if it worked so well, why come off at all?

Because that's not food freedom.

By staying on your reset, you'll miss the opportunity to enjoy some truly special, truly significant, truly delicious foods. (Think: your gram's baklava, that bottle of red you picked up on your honeymoon, or the warm biscuits with butter and jam at your favorite restaurant.) You'll miss the opportunity to build confidence by turning down foods you've decided aren't worth it, but saying yes to things you really love and want to experience. And you won't expand your diet to include the broadest range of foods while staying in control and feeling your best.

You don't want to limit yourself to your reset foods forever. It's time to figure out how much wiggle room you have—how much you can "get away with" while still remaining confident in your food choices, feeling as energetic, happy, and healthy as you want.

It's time to learn how to ride your new bike.

STEP 2:
ENJOYING FOOD FREEDOM

- Make conscious, deliberate decisions to eat less-healthy foods
- Eat only as much as you need to satisfy the experience
- Savor thoughtfully, without guilt, shame, or remorse
- Return to normal, healthy habits

Step 2 in the Food Freedom plan is taking what you learned from your reset and applying it in the real world in a conscious, deliberate fashion; crafting and enjoying the perfect, sustainable diet for you. Your goal is to have as few self-imposed restrictions as possible while still retaining all (or most) of the benefits you gained during your reset. Food freedom looks different from your reset for a number of reasons, including this one:

You will only restrict things if *you* decide they aren't worth it.

Think of it this way: If someone told you that you could have a chocolate chip cookie and a glass of wine every day and still feel energetic and well rested, wouldn't you want to do that? If it were possible to bookend dinner with fresh-from-the-oven rolls and ice cream without your cravings and waistline rebelling, you'd be all over that, right? Shoot, you'd do a happy dance if you could just add some cream back into your morning coffee without any stomach gurgles or congestion.

Post-reintroduction, your ideal food freedom diet should immediately expand based on what you learned. There will be things you reincorporate that make you supremely happy with zero negative consequences. Maybe the added sugar in your favorite maple chicken sausage is no big deal, half-and-half in your coffee doesn't upset your stomach, and the white rice on your sushi doesn't hurt your energy levels. GREAT. This is a major win-win, and there is no reason you shouldn't bring these things back into your regular diet. Just make sure your breakfast tastes don't keep growing sweeter and sweeter, your coffee consumption doesn't creep into long-distance-trucker territory as a result of your new cream habit, and your energy truly isn't suffering with the return of your beloved sushi three nights in a row. Step 2 is also about slowly and carefully figuring out your tipping point—how far, how often, and with which foods can you stray off-course before the negative consequences of those choices are no longer acceptable to you?

You still need to pay attention.

Your perfect food freedom diet should also include some foods that you know make you less healthy. Yeah, you heard me: the meals that have cultural significance, the foods that only come around once a year (see: chocolate crème eggs), that cake your mom makes with a cup of Crisco (A CUP) but you can't imagine turning it down, the stuff you decide is so incredibly delicious that it's worth the health consequences . . . *you should eat those things, too.* The trick is figuring out how, in a way that satisfies but doesn't send you off the rails with your health or self-control.

Is It Worth It? Let Me Work It.

This starts with your own personal decisions about "worth it" foods and drinks. You'll hear this phrase so often throughout the book that it's worth defining: "Worth it" is anything you know will likely have negative physical or psychological consequences, but is so special, enjoyable, or significant that you choose to eat it anyway.

The key to "worth it" is that you have to decide this for yourself—I can't do it for you. (That's also very good news, because someone else making decisions for you isn't exactly "freedom.") The bowl of ice cream that you know, thanks to reintroduction, will make your skin break out—is that worth it? Maybe it is, because you love ice cream that much. Good for you! Enjoy, and deal with the consequence. Maybe it's not, because maintaining clear skin is way more important than five minutes of creamy, cold happiness. That's all good, too. The key is making the decisions and holding yourself accountable; declining when you decide something just *isn't* worth it, even if it's tempting.

You already have a good idea about "worth it" foods and beverages based on your reintroduction experience. If you reintroduced something and it went horribly wrong (digestive distress, energy disruptions, pain or inflammation, a return of symptoms), it's probably safe to assume you'll be leaving that food out of your general Food Freedom plan. For me, this is goat cheese. That particular cheese makes me feel like that guy on the gurney in the first *Alien* movie—the one who has that creepy worm thing unceremoniously burst out of his body. For that reason, it's never worth it, and I'll go out of my way to ensure I'm not accidentally exposed to it in a salad or appetizer. Even if the Pope himself offered me goat cheese, I would politely say, "No, thank you, your Holiness," but I wouldn't tell him why, because holy TMI.

WORTH IT, EXPANDED

Worth it" isn't just about the physical consequences; it's also about evaluating how a particular food affects your brain, your emotional attachment to other foods, your willpower, and your cravings. Some foods won't impact your energy, sleep, or digestion, but they'll leave you craving sugar or carbs like crazy; for example, many Whole30ers report that eating something salty automatically makes them want something sweet. You may discover that other foods (or drinks—I'm looking at you, alcohol) are "gateway foods," bringing to mind associations or past experiences that make you automatically reach for other less-healthy foods. Some foods may impact you in both ways; gluten (if you're sensitive to it) can contribute to both digestive distress and mental health conditions like depression and seasonal affective disorder. The emotional and psychological side effects of eating these potentially less-healthy foods are just as significant as the physical consequences, so make sure you take them into account during your "worth it" evaluations.

Here's the rub: The reintroduction period alone won't tell you everything you need to know to make accurate "worth it" decisions. You'll gain some big-picture ideas of how food affects you during reintroduction, and that's good. But factors like dose, frequency, and variety all matter. You may feel different eating two slices of toast at breakfast versus half a piece. You may feel okay eating a yogurt one day, but eating one three days in a row makes you bloated and wheezy. You may do well with hard cheeses, but soft cheeses bring digestive distress.

It's impossible to account for all these scenarios during the set reintroduction period, which brings you to an important food freedom lesson:

Reintroduction is a lifelong practice.

Every time you eat a potentially problematic food, you have to pay attention to how it makes you feel and compare that to your baseline: how awesome you felt after your reset. Every. Single. Time. This means no mindless consumption, no automatic decision-making, no deliberately shutting off your brain ("I'm not going to worry about it tonight—I'm just going to eat whatever I want!"). Food freedom demands that you pay better attention than that. But it's also not as hard as it sounds, and it gets easier with practice.

Conscious and Deliberate

Here's how it works: You go about your days eating the post-reset diet you've decided works best for you, feeling awesome and in control. This diet looks broader than your reset and is way more sustainable, because you've relaxed on certain ingredients (like the maple in your chicken sausage) and brought back some things you've missed (like white rice) based on what you learned during reintroduction. Then, something outside of your "norm" pops up; something so special, delicious, or significant that you don't think you want to pass up.

Start by asking yourself the most important questions: Is this worth it? Is the taste or experience going to be so good that it makes up for the potential negative health consequences? Will it mess you up not at all, for a little while, or for a long time? (Use your best judgment here—you won't always know for sure.) Take what you learned during reintroduction and imagine those consequences as completely as possible, factoring in physical, emotional, and psychological effects. One glass of wine may not upset your stomach or impact your energy, but it may leave you uninhibited enough to order the nacho cheese fries, which are decidedly *not* worth it, along with another glass.

Part of the "worth it" evaluation is also asking yourself, do I really want it? If might be your favorite food of all time, and totally worth it based on past experiences, but you're just not feeling it today (like my birthday and the cupcake). It's important to honor your truth in that moment by asking yourself if you even want it in the first place, and declining if you relaize you just don't. (Nothing derails food freedom faster than eating something you knew you didn't really want, leaving you feeling out of control and disappointed in yourself.)

SOCIAL GRACES

Sometimes, this decision will be less about the food itself and more about the experience. You should take that into account, too. If I'm at a wedding, I usually toast the bride and groom with sparkling water, because that feels just as festive to me as raising a glass of champagne, and unless it's my favorite brand, champagne isn't worth it. But when I'm at my sister's Thanksgiving dinner and everyone is passing a bottle of wine, taking a sip and saying what they're grateful for, I want to fully participate in that experience. It's not about the wine—it's about the social interaction and the good feelings that tradition bring. For me, that's well worth the health consequences of a big swig of booze—and the germs I'm sharing with the 12 people who drank straight from the bottle before me. If you're Catholic, this should not faze you.

News flash: Food freedom also means considering any alternatives that will satisfy you without the negative consequences. Family dinner might be just as great if you talk over a cup of herbal tea while everyone else eats dessert. Happy hours can be just as happy with sparkling water and lime in your glass. Bring coconut milk ice cream to your company's picnic if that will allow you to build your own sundae without the bloat.

You should also ask yourself, Do I need to eat or drink anything at all to satisfy this experience? You *can* celebrate someone's birthday without cake. Like, it's physically possible. You should explore those options, too.

Finally, ask yourself again: Is this worth it? Yes, this question is *that* important, but you're also buying yourself some time here. In the moment, when the reward is right in front of you and your brain is screaming for it, you're going to want to make an impulse decision for instant gratification. Getting into the habit of pausing and asking yourself these questions before you automatically indulge will help you stay in control and avoid the regret that comes with eating something you don't really want.

And now it's time for a reality check.

While this all sounds *delightful*, there's also a really good chance that these concepts are so foreign to you that you'll have a hard time putting them into actual practice. You're probably conditioned to turn off conscious decision-making when faced with a rewarding food or automatically justify its consumption without actually considering whether you even want it. It's going to take practice to willfully override that habit, so you can focus on asking yourself all the "worth it" questions necessary to make the right decision in the moment.

LESS BAD ISN'T ALWAYS GOOD

You may be tempted to automatically choose the "healthier" option when considering an off-plan treat, like a gluten-free beer versus your beloved Guinness, or an almond flour muffin instead of the corner bakery version you really want, but that may not always be your most worth-it option. These gluten-free, naturally sweetened, alternative-flour recreations aren't necessarily healthier; they're just less bad. But if you don't enjoy them anywhere near as much as the real deal, is that really a wiser choice? You're still eating something that makes you less healthy, you're still pushing more nutritious food off your plate, and you're not even enjoying it that much—which actually sounds like a net loss. The lesson? Sometimes, eating the real thing (and suffering the consequences) is actually a *better* choice than opting for the less delicious, less bad option.

This is a new skill, and you're not going to be good at it right away.

It's going to feel like hard work at first. You may not even remember to switch gears until after the first bite. You will probably still find yourself automatically accepting the offer of rewarding foods out of sheer habit. This is okay. The key is not to panic, or think you've blown it, or beat yourself up about it. And I certainly don't want you to think, "Oh, well" and eat your way through the rest of the pantry.

You don't do that anymore.

You will learn how to create this new relationship with food. And in this next chapter, I'll hand over an arsenal of tools to help.

AS PART OF YOUR FOOD FREEDOM PLAN, ASK YOURSELF THESE QUESTIONS BEFORE CONSUMING A POTENTIALLY LESS-HEALTHY FOOD OR BEVERAGE.

- Is it worth it?

- Is the taste or experience worth the potential negative consequences?

- How will consuming this impact me physically, mentally, or emotionally?

- Will it "mess me up" not at all, a little, or significantly?

- Do I really want it?

- Is there a "less bad" alternative that will satisfy me just as much?

- Do I need to consume anything here to enjoy the experience?

- Is it worth it?

CHAPTER 7

IN-THE-MOMENT SUCCESS STRATEGIES

Just like any other skill, there's a learning curve to food freedom. Creating new habits will require commitment and practice before they start feeling effortless. However, changing a habit is a lot easier when you have the right tools at your disposal, and there are four techniques straight out of habit, stress, and willpower research that can buy you the time, space, and distance you'll need to practice good decision-making. Pick one, or combine them all for maximum effectiveness.

Note, however, that the goal here *isn't* to resist at all costs; it's simply to make the right decision for you in that moment. Now that your reset is over, there is no need to arbitrarily deny yourself a delicious, special, worth-it treat, even if it happens to be spectacularly unhealthy. That's old dieting mentality, and only leads to the same yo-yo pattern you've been stuck in for years: resist, resist, resist . . . binge. These tools aren't supposed to help you say no—they're supposed to help you wait, evaluate, then decide based on what is right for you in that moment.

DEEP BREATHS: This one is so simple, and yet so effective. When faced with temptation, your brain releases dopamine, a neurotransmitter responsible for your motivation to pursue a specific rewarding behavior. Dopamine does not provide happiness, only the promise of happiness. And when dopamine has your attention, you become fixated on that reward. (To keep things simple, you can think of dopamine as your Sugar Dragon, breathing fire and insisting you do as you're told while promising delicious bliss and immediate satisfaction.)

This is also perceived by the body as stress, which is why you feel anxious and slightly out of control thinking about your treat. "Am I going to eat it? Should I eat it? I probably shouldn't . . . but I probably will." In the face of this stress, your breathing also changes to a stressful breath pattern—it becomes more shallow, faster, and takes place higher up in the chest. Kind of like panic breathing.

There is no need to panic here. It's just a cupcake.

By changing your breathing pattern, you can send a signal to your nervous system that you're actually DOING JUST FINE, which helps you activate the willpower center of your brain and feel more in control. Practice slowing your breathing down to a 2:1 ratio of exhale to inhale (like an eight-count exhale followed by a four-count inhale), and breathe into your diaphragm; this is known as belly breathing. You can practice this throughout the day, and put it into immediate effect when faced with a decision to eat something you know makes you less healthy. It may sound like voodoo, but deep breathing has been successfully used by U.S. soldiers, Hurricane Katrina survivors, and kids being cyberbullied; it will probably help with your cupcake. (For other stress-relieving breathing techniques, do an Internet search for "tactical breathing" or "4-7-8 breathing.")

"I CAN HAVE IT LATER": Temptation overwhelms you the most when the reward is immediately available and staring you in the face. To combat this effect, put that food or drink in a brief time-out.

Institute a 15-minute, 1-hour, or 1-day waiting period; whatever feels appropriate. Tell yourself you're not going to eat it now, but if you still really want it 15 minutes from now (or an hour from now, or tomorrow), you'll allow yourself to enjoy it then. This gives your brain the space it needs to evaluate whether you truly want it, whether you're just feeling bored/anxious/lonely, etc., and whether or not it will actually be worth it. Employ this waiting period every time you're faced with a potentially worth-it food. Even if you only give yourself until the waiter comes back, removing or delaying the possibility of "right now" will help relieve some of the pressure.

EMPLOY DISTRACTION: In Walter Mischel's famous "Marshmallow Test" from 1960, four- to six-year-olds' willpower was tested using marshmallows as a reward. The children who were successfully able to delay gratification (the joy of eating one marshmallow placed right in front of them) for a bigger reward (two marshmallows to eat when the experiment was over) succeeded by employing a variety of distraction techniques. Some covered their eyes, some turned their backs on the tempting marshmallow, and others sang to themselves.

While you probably shouldn't start belting out Taylor Swift when they roll out the donuts at your business meeting, you can employ similar distraction techniques when you have an unexpected encounter with tempting food. Remove yourself from the temptation by closing the dessert menu, leaving the break room, or moving the chips and salsa out of your immediate reach. Tell a story to shift the focus of the room off the treats, engage with someone next to you, or start taking meticulous meeting notes (scoring bonus points with your boss in the process).

USE YOUR IMAGINATION: You can also harness the power of imagination to help you decide. Studies find that trying not to think about a particular food (like chocolate) only makes you want it more, but imagining the consumption of that food can actually decrease your appetite for it. You can take that a step further by thinking about how you'll feel later in the day if you do choose to indulge. Do you know from experience that you'll be mad at yourself for giving in when you know darn well it's not worth it? Can you see yourself running to the bathroom all day, something you can't afford with your big presentation coming up? Will you get home too lethargic to play with your kids, knowing you promised them you'd go to the park before dinner? Those are all strikes against the indulgence. However, if you picture yourself feeling not quite as awesome but still happy you decided to go for it, that's a pretty good indication of "worth it."

One trick I use is telling myself the opposite of what I think I want, and then evaluating how I feel about it: I'll pretend that someone just told me, "Oops, sorry. There aren't any cupcakes left." If I feel indifferent or relieved, then I know this is a food I can skip. If I get super-bummed, that tells me this may be a treat worth indulging in. Little tricks like this only take a mental moment, and can all help you get to the root of the questions "Is it worth it?" and "Do I really want it?"

Using one or more of these strategies when faced with a delicious treat means your Sugar Dragon is less likely to automatically win this round, and should buy you the time, space, and mental energy to decide whether that food or drink is really worth it for you. If you decide it's not, you can move on down the road without feeling deprived, because *you* were the one who chose not to indulge. If you decide it is worth it, yay! But before you take that first bite . . .

Food freedom thinks we should talk about it *just* a little bit more first. Just tell your treat to wait for like, five more minutes.

When You Indulge

So let's recap: You're eating your post-reintroduction food freedom diet, and something amazingly delicious (and spectacularly unhealthy) comes your way—say, a peanut butter chocolate chip vanilla frosted cookie. You run through your checklist, and create the distance and space you need to accurately evaluate whether it's actually worth it, and whether you actually want it. (It is, and you do!) You accept the delicious treat and consciously, deliberately take your first bite. From here, this experience could go one of two ways.

The first way: It tastes like vanilla-frosted rainbows (or just meh, but you convince yourself otherwise), and since you've already started to eat it, you might as well finish it. You consume the rest quickly and excitedly, your brain exploding with joy as you cram it into your face-hole. In this instance, the treat is gone before you even realize it, you barely got to enjoy the experience, and your brain is already screaming for more.

Please don't do that.

To make the most out of this experience, to really make the potential health consequences worth it . . .

You have to savor it.

Take your time. Pay attention to the taste, flavor, texture. Create the kind of environment that will allow you to enjoy what you're eating. Get downright romantic with that cookie. This starts with the very first bite.

It might stop with the very first bite, too.

THE ONE-BITE RULE: Here's a bonus in-the-moment success strategy you may find helpful: If you think your less-healthy treat is going to be so delicious, so incredible, so worth it . . . and then you take your first bite and discover it's not, STOP EATING. (I call this "Melissa's One-Bite Rule," in existence since the infamous Portland Donut Incident of 2015. The summary: Everyone promised it would be orgasmic, but it was just okay—SORRY, CITY OF PORTLAND.)

The only reason to indulge in a less-healthy treat in the first place is if it's so incredibly, deliriously worth it that you're willing to accept the less-healthy consequences. So if you discover it's not what you imagined, why keep eating? (It's not like it's good for you, after all.) If the black-and-white rules of your reset really worked for you, create a hard-and-fast rule for this, too. "Every time I eat a less-healthy food, the One-Bite Rule goes into effect." That helps to take some of the effort of decision-making out of your hands and keeps you from that icky feeling you get while continuing to eat something unhealthy that's not even that good.

CLEAN YOUR PLATE?

Many of you have been conditioned not to waste food. I was raised with a "clear your plate" mentality, too, so I get it. Do your best to prevent this dilemma in the first place. Help yourself to just a tiny serving to begin with, take a bite of a friend's dish first, or ask the waiter for a taste before you order a full glass. But if you do get partway through something and realize you don't want the rest, you'll have to ask yourself what's more important: maintaining your health, self-confidence, and sense of control around food, or not throwing out half a cookie you've already paid for? In that moment, I will always encourage you to stop eating. Always. This is your *health*, and eating the rest of that cookie isn't going to benefit your local homeless shelter anyway. If you end up with something you don't actually want, see if a friend or co-worker wants the rest, or bring it home for your roommates. But wrap your head around the idea that throwing the rest away may be the best decision for you—and that you don't need to punish yourself for a bad judgment call by sacrificing your own health.

If that first bite is as delicious as you had hoped, fantastic! Give yourself a minute to truly appreciate what you're eating, pausing to take part in the social interaction, or simply taking a quiet moment by yourself to be happy with what's on your plate. Then take your second bite . . . and repeat the process. Is the second bite as good as the first? Is it still worth it? Is this bite enough to make you feel satisfied with the experience?

Continue with this evaluation until you've decided you are satisfied with the flavor, the food, or the experience. Maybe this is half a cookie. Maybe this is three cookies. Both are okay, as long as every bite is conscious, deliberate, and worth it.

Here's where it gets tricky: Every time you're faced with a new social dynamic, a new situation, or a new combination of ingredients, you have to evaluate all over again, taking your environment, emotional state, and health goals into consideration. Just because that famous-brand donut was worth it yesterday morning doesn't mean it will still be worth it this morning. If you enjoyed gluten-free toast with breakfast last week, that doesn't mean you'll want to do it every week. Your context changes. Your goals change. Your health changes. That means what's worth it will also always be changing.

Every time you have the opportunity to enjoy a potentially less-healthy food, you have to reevaluate whether or not it's worth it. I'll illustrate with a story: I generally avoid gluten, because if I eat too much, my belly gets so bloated people start asking when I'm due. During the last holiday season, I indulged more than usual, because I came across lots of once-a-year, totally-worth-it baked treats, and I didn't mind being a little bloated under my stretchy jeans. But in February before my Costa Rica yoga retreat, I declined all gluten, even if the treat was incredibly tempting or special, because I knew I'd be in formfitting yoga clothes and I wanted to look my best.

Vanity is a perfectly acceptable reason for declining a less-healthy treat.

My point is this: You should *always* be paying attention, *always* evaluating "worth it" potential, and *always* making conscious, deliberate decisions when considering a less-healthy food. That's the kind of attentiveness that food freedom demands.

Oh, but this time, it will actually work.

Yes, every other diet in the world tells you to "eat mindfully" and "listen to your body." And no, that's never actually worked for you before. But remember, this time, you didn't diet, you *reset*. You changed your blood sugar regulation, hormonal balance, and taste buds, so you can trust the signals your body is sending you. You tamed your Sugar Dragon, reduced or eliminated cravings, and regained control of your food choices. You remained well fed and well nourished, so there's no physiological urge to rebound by eating All the Things. You're now totally set up to actually eat mindfully and truly listen to your body. And for the first time in a long time, your body is no longer lying to you.

Given that this is your new context, you really *can* listen and pay attention every time you eat something less healthy.

TAKE A PAUSE

A nother trick that may help in the moment: Make a habit of putting down your fork or glass between every bite or sip. This gives you a physical cue to think about what you're eating and how it's making you feel. It also buys your digestive tract some time to send the signal to your brain that you're full or satisfied. (True story: There is a product called the HAPIfork that measures your time between bites and vibrates if you're eating too quickly. It also connects with your smartphone via Bluetooth, transmitting statistics like "fork servings" and intervals between bites. Or, you know, you could just save yourself the $79 and stop eating like you're in prison.)

On paper, this may sound like overkill: tedious and artificial, like you're psychoanalyzing everything you put in your mouth. But in practice, this is actually the process that keeps you *connected* to what you're eating, feeling in control and listening to the signals your body is sending you. It may be hard to follow this strategy perfectly in every situation; sometimes you're eating the cake while standing up, minding your toddler, and trying to carry on a conversation with your friend. But that doesn't give you an excuse to mindlessly hoover whatever sweet treat is on your plate.

I have been known to say to my toddler, "Hold on, love. Mama's taking a bite of her peanut butter cup."

The Language of Food

Over time and with practice, you'll learn to reconnect (and stay connected) to your food using these techniques, which will help you feel like you're always in control of what you're eating. This is also the key to eliminating feelings of guilt or shame around your food choices. Wait, let me say that again, because it's really important.

**Eliminate "guilt" and "shame" from
your food vocabulary.**

Food freedom catalyzes you to change your relationship with food. It also requires you to take an honest look at one more aspect of your life-changing transformation: your vocabulary.

Negative self-talk is one of the fastest ways of destroying self-esteem, sabotaging your goals, and upsetting your mood and emotions. "Fat-talk" (speaking disapprovingly about your body) can lead to body dysmorphia, disordered eating habits, and low self-esteem. Statements like "I could have," "I should be," and "I used to" short-circuit progress toward your goals, and keep you focused on the past or future, not your accomplishments here in the present. But what about the words you use to describe your food choices?

"I was so good today; I ate really healthy."

"I was so bad today! I had ice cream and cake at the party."

"I cheated on my diet with a glass of wine."

"I totally failed—there were bread crumbs in that dish."

"I've been behaving with my diet; no gluten or dairy."

"I'm a disaster—I can't stop eating sugar."

The words you choose to describe your food and yourself have real power. Treating yourself like a child who needs to "be good" on their diet is misguided. What happens when a child misbehaves? They are punished. Food should never be associated with punishment. Imagining your diet as a jealous lover who will be critical and disapproving if you "cheat" is damaging. Feeling guilt and shame over your "infidelities" will never lead to true food freedom. Linking your food choices with your "success" or "failure" as a person is destructive. Who you are and your self-worth has nothing to do with the potato chips or broccoli on your plate.

Insulting yourself for your choices—any choices—is perhaps the most harmful behavior of all. You aren't a mess, a disaster, or a train wreck. You aren't hopeless, worthless, or pathetic. You are a committed, motivated, healthy person working hard to change your relationship with food, grappling with strong emotional ties and the pull of long-standing habits. You are so much more than the results of your struggles.

Someone asked me on Facebook recently, "I ate a Whole30-inspired diet all day, and I know what to call that—I just say I ate Whole30. But what should I call it when later, I eat some pizza? Cheat? Slip? Fail?"

What if you just called it "eating pizza"?

As you change your relationship with food through this program, I invite you to develop a new language around your food. You are not good or bad based on your choices. They are simply choices.

You do not cheat; you make a choice.

You do not fail; you make a choice.

Your choices do not define you as a person.

There is no guilt, shame, or punishment, only consequence.

Imagine, for a moment, that your food is just food, and that your choices are just choices. What you eat is not a statement about your self-worth, your value, or your significance in this world.

Believe this, and everything changes.

You used to feel guilty about the treats you ate because it felt like you were "cheating" on your diet, or you mindlessly ate it up so fast it barely registered, or you lost control and overconsumed, giving in to cravings and eating things you didn't even want to eat. But this is not that. Here, you are consciously and deliberately choosing to include this "worth it" food in your diet—it's a choice, not a cheat. Here, you are savoring each morsel, allowing yourself to enjoy the taste and texture and appreciate the pleasure it brings. Here, you are making a conscious, deliberate decision with every single bite, eating only as much as you need to satisfy the experience; stopping when you decide you've had enough, not because you're stuffed and feeling sick.

As part of your food freedom, "guilt" and "shame" are no longer words in your food vocabulary. There is no guilt, only consequences, and you're not doing anything wrong. In fact, just the opposite, because you're making educated decisions that are uniquely right for you. Isn't that refreshing?

This practice will also minimize most of your post-consumption regret, something that used to happen every time you indulged.

Most, but not all.

Regret Is Inevitable

Occasionally, you'll make a conscious, deliberate decision to indulge; confirm every bite is worth it; stop when you've satisfied the experience . . . and sometime later, realize you've made a horrible mistake. You experience stomach pain or digestive distress, your energy plummets, your cravings return with a vengeance, or your joints become swollen. When all is said and done, you think, "Well *that* wasn't worth it at all."

If this catches you by surprise, this experience can derail you from your food freedom track because it feels a like failure. You made the wrong decision, and chose poorly. You feel like crap as a result. You think all the good work you've put in has been erased with one bad choice. You consider the experience a giant crash-and-burn, and beat yourself up about it for the rest of the day. Or week. Or month. And you know where *that* leads—a reckless return to Carb-a-Palooza, because you've messed it all up and what's the point, anyway?

Stop and reframe. *You haven't failed.* You actually followed your plan to the letter; a win in and of itself! But some regret is inevitable.

How else are you supposed to learn?

Remember, reintroduction is a lifelong process. While it would be lovely if you were able to accurately predict how everything you eat will impact you, in practice, that's impossible. The only way to know for sure is to try, and sometimes, it will not go well. This isn't a failure—it's actually a really valuable teaching tool. Now you get to log the experience in your notebook (mental or otherwise) and add it to your evaluations of "worth it" or "not worth it" in future situations, making you more effective at accurately predicting the consequences of future off-plan indulgences.

An experiment gone wrong is no longer a failure—it's a learning experience ... which means there is no reason to beat yourself up, punish yourself, or comfort yourself with more less-healthy food. This is such an important concept, and one that's probably totally new. I promise, if you can truly pick up what I'm putting down here, it will make all the difference.

Having said that, I'll also acknowledge that your brain can be a stubborn brat, and you may need to learn your lesson the hard way more than once.

That's how it was with me and gluten-free toast. Every time I ordered it, I thought, "This time, the toast will be delicious and worth it." And every single time, it just wasn't tasty. More like damp cardboard. Not at all worth it. Still, I persisted, because I was hopeful I'd find a delicious toast option that I could eat occasionally without the effects of gluten. But every time, I'd take a bite and say, "Oh, that's why I never order this."

My brain still plays tricks on me, too.

The difference is that now, when I order something that isn't worth it, I don't finish it just because I told myself I could; instead, I pawn it off on friends who do enjoy it. I don't get mad at myself for making the wrong choice; I tell myself, "Remember this for next time," and ask the waitress for a side of mixed berries instead. I don't eat everything else in sight because I've already "ruined" my diet for the day. That's old diet-think, and I've left all that behind. (P.S. Eventually, this particular lesson stuck. Now I no longer order gluten-free toast, and if I want the flavor and texture of toast that much, I order the sourdough and accept the consequences.)

If you find yourself reliving the same lesson again and again, don't be discouraged. You're trying to overwrite decades of habits and associations, and the brain really likes to be rewarded (even if your taste buds aren't that jazzed about it). Be patient, and be persistent. The day will come when that lesson will click just like it did for me, and you'll have yet another milestone to celebrate on your food freedom path.

We Now Return to Your Regularly Scheduled Diet

The final part of enjoying your food freedom is returning right back to your regularly scheduled diet as soon as your indulgence is over. This is called Avoiding the "What the Hell" Effect, and yes, that is a legitimate psychological term. Okay, willpower expert Roy Baumeister says this is technically called counter-regulatory eating, but the slang is catchy, right? Also, I'm pretty sure you already know what this is.

You give in to a craving, deviating from your normal diet to enjoy a treat. As soon as you do, your brain tries to persuade you that all is already lost (your health, waistline, and willpower), so you might as well eat All the Things. It's the dietary equivalent of making a detour for gas on your way to study at the library, then saying, "What the hell, I'm already off course" and driving to Vegas instead.

Hey, if you're going to fail, you might as well fail spectacularly.

Happily, there is far less room for your brain to invoke the WTH Effect in your Food Freedom plan. You're making conscious decisions to eat something less healthy because you've decided it's worth it. You are fully aware of how this food is likely to impact you, physically and psychologically. You eat mindfully, savoring the experience and stopping when you're satisfied. You experience no guilt or shame, because you made a deliberate choice, and you don't think about food like that anymore. And because you haven't been starving yourself or arbitrarily restricting, you feel less physiological pull to overconsume sugar or carbs.

So you eat, enjoy, deal with the consequences, and go right back to your new, healthful way of eating. You stay there until the next time something special, significant, or delicious comes across your plate, when you repeat the entire process; from asking, "Is this worth it?" to returning to your normal, healthy eating plan.

That's it. Simple, right?

Sometimes, an amazing food or drink will enter your field of vision five times a day, like if you're on vacation in Napa. Sometimes, an entire week will go by where it turns out nothing you encounter is actually special or tasty enough to indulge in. Either way, as long as you're following the plan, you'll continue to stay in control and generally feel awesome . . . once the effect of all that zinfandel wears off.

Now, another reality check.

Despite your best-laid plans and all the tips I've provided thus far, from time to time you're still going to ride the struggle-bus down Food Freedom Road. Staying conscientious, making sure it's worth it, and retaining control in today's busy, stressful world is hard. Overriding decades of habits, associations, and behaviors around less-healthy foods is really hard. Trying to implement your new Food Freedom plan when that cute bartender in Mexico sends your whole group a round of poolside tequila shots is COME ON NOW THAT'S NOT EVEN FAIR.

NO CHEAT DAYS

The idea of a "cheat day" flies in the face of food freedom. First, think about what you'll want to eat for dinner next Tuesday. Wait—you have no idea, because that's days from now, and how are you supposed to know what you'll be in the mood for? The same principle applies to sweets and treats. How do you know you're going to want to eat French fries, cookies, and candy on Sunday? You won't, until it's Sunday and you evaluate these foods individually and deliberately in the moment. But if you tell yourself you *can* have them, on Sunday morning, the plane is landing all over again—reward is on the horizon; let the uncontrollable cravings commence. You can't plan for worth-it foods, even if you know you've got something potentially tempting on the horizon. Until you arrive at your birthday dinner and are face-to-face with the dessert menu, you can't accurately evaluate whether, *in that moment*, the cake is worth it or not. The lesson? There are no cheat days when you're enjoying food freedom, because if everything is a careful, conscious decision, there is absolutely nothing to cheat *on*.

I wish I could say, "Just do this!" and provide you with a magical trick to keep you on track. Unfortunately, there is no one universal tip that will work to keep everyone on the right path equally well. The key to making lasting changes is having plenty of tools in your toolbox, and pulling them out one by one when you need them until you figure out which is right for the particular job.

First, gather lots of coping strategies—as many as you can think of. Write them all down, because in the heat of the moment, you may come up blank when trying to recall them. Then, when tempted with a rewarding food (especially in the face of stress or other emotions), run through your list, on paper or in your head. Choose a strategy that seems applicable to your current situation. Try it.

Did it work? Sweet! You're one step further in your food freedom journey. Did it not work? NO PROBLEM—pick another strategy. Try that one, too. Did it work? Success! If not, keep running down your list, pulling out as many different tools as you need to get you through the moment while staying true to your long-term goal. Remember:

**Your goal is *not* to avoid eating
the delicious treat.**

Your goal is to conscientiously evaluate whether it's worth it and you want it, and make the decision that's right for you in the moment. Maybe that's eating the food. Maybe that's passing. Either way, what's important is that it's a deliberate decision, and not an involuntary snap judgment based on impulse, habit, or emotion.

I've already given you some effective tools, taken straight out of habit and willpower research. (Feel free to add to this list based on successful in-the-moment strategies that have worked for you in the past.)

- **Calming breathing techniques**

- **Creating temporal distance ("I can have it in fifteen minutes/ one hour/one day.")**

- **Employing distraction**

- **Using your imagination**

- **Enacting the One-Bite Rule**

- **Pausing between sips or bites**

These quick tactics can be used right in the moment to help you make good choices when temptation looms. However, there are also some big-picture practices you can implement to maintain your hard-earned food freedom. Let's talk about those next.

CHAPTER 8

BIG-PICTURE FOOD FREEDOM SUCCESS STRATEGIES

For the last several chapters, you've been happily skipping hand in hand with food freedom, learning how to enjoy not-so-healthy-but-still-worth-it foods while feeling totally in control. You've tasted—then tossed—half a cookie that wasn't that good, savored two glasses of wine that were really good, and are still deciding whether that birthday cake is going to be worth it. (You've been thinking about it too long, which means it's probably not.) Once your delicious treat is over, you go right back to your normal, healthy diet, easy-peasy.

Except that sometimes, it doesn't feel easy. Or peasy.

You can use all of your tools effectively, treating yo'self only when it's really worth it, then getting back to your normal, healthy diet right on schedule . . . but still feel like you're just barely hanging on to your food freedom. Like the next sugary, salty, fatty thing to come your way could be the tipping point that sends you running right back to old habits. Like if you have to deep-breathe in a business meeting *one more time*, you'll probably hyperventilate that donut right into your mouth.

First, please know that this is totally normal. Second, it will get better and easier fast. Third, there are more tricks up my sleeve, and I'm about to share them all with you.

The in-the-moment success strategies from chapter 8 are like a temporary patch; useful right then and there to help you achieve your goal. But they're not long-term solutions, because eventually it would be nice to not have to breathe, wait, distract, and imagine every time you're face-to-face with a potato chip. Ideally you'll be able to process the opportunity quickly and efficiently, responding with a decisive "Yes, please" or "No, thank you" right on the spot—and getting the "Is it worth it?" question right far more times than not.

To get there, you'll need more than just a temporary patch; you'll need some big-picture interventions designed to rewire your body and brain to be better at food freedoming.

Yeah, I just made that a verb.

Growth Mind-set

The first incredibly helpful trick is reframing your perspective from a fixed mind-set to a growth mind-set. What's the difference? A fixed mind-set means you believe your traits or qualities are stuck, unable to be changed or improved. This is you if you can remember, with crystal clarity, your mom saying, "He's going to be husky" or "She's going to have my hips" and still seeing a husky/hippy person in the mirror, no matter what you weigh now. This is you if, having been told as a kid that you weren't athletic, you never tried out for a sport and to this day won't accept a co-worker's invitation to play pick-up basketball. A fixed mind-set makes you believe your health, athletic abilities, intelligence, or other key traits don't change as you move through life; they just are what they are.

A fixed mind-set will hold you back when it comes to embracing food freedom.

If you've long considered yourself unhealthy—if you've been over-weight, sedentary, sick, or hooked on junk food for most of your adult life—a fixed mind-set will tell you that you'll always be an unhealthy person. Even if you do lose weight or change your diet, your Debbie Downer brain will keep reminding you that you're not *really* healthy, because you're stuck with the health status you assigned yourself years ago.

It's going to be impossible to create new, lasting, healthy habits if you believe you can't really change.

The best thing you can do for your Food Freedom plan is to adopt a growth mind-set, as I did when I was first out of rehabilitation and working hard to stay clean. With a growth mind-set, you believe traits are malleable; able to develop and improve with commitment and effort. There are neuro-physiological benefits to a growth mind-set, too—which is just a fancy way of saying that with a growth mind-set, your brain also gets better at recog-nizing and learning from missteps. If this was your way of thinking, you'd be motivated to get stronger and more coordinated so you could join that basketball team, change your study tactics to improve your grades, and . . .

Label yourself as a healthy person.

Adopting a growth mind-set as part of your initial reset can make a huge dif-ference in your commitment, motivation, and effort. Starting on Day 1, make your mantra "I am a healthy person, living a healthy lifestyle." Find ways to demonstrate to yourself how that's true. Keep a journal of what you're doing to take good care of yourself; revisit your Non-Scale Victory checklist (page 33) to see what's improving; place sticky notes with growth mind-set rein-forcement around the house, and every time you find yourself back in a fixed mind-set, thinking, "This will never change" or "I always give up," reframe your perspective with a mantra that works for you.

Maybe that's "I'm a Food Freedom badass," which gets a thumbs-up from me.

There's also another language trick you can use here, straight out of habit research. Instead of labeling your behaviors as healthy, committed, or motivated, label *yourself* as those things.

INSTEAD OF: "I eat a healthy diet."

TRY: "I am a healthy eater."

These might sound the same to you, but attaching desirable character-istics to yourself instead of your actions makes you more likely to model those behaviors. In one example, students who practiced the mantra "I do not cheat on tests" were more likely to cheat when given the opportunity than those who practiced saying, "I am not a cheater." The act of attaching the desired behavior to you as a person solidifies it in your brain, helping you maintain your commitment, even in times of stress.

You can apply that research to other areas of your life by changing your internal dialogue around the habits you're trying to enforce. Think, "I am an exerciser," instead of "I like exercise"; or "I am a self-motivated person" instead of "I will keep up my motivation." The more you can embody these traits in your actions, words, and thoughts, the more likely they are to stick.

SEEK GROWTH

Having a hard time getting into a growth mind-set? Find examples in your own life where you've already proven it true. Think back to a time when someone told you (or you told yourself), "You can't do that" or "You're not good at that," but you got better by working hard. These examples can be small; a task at the office, an instrument you played as a kid, a social skill you developed, a class in which you improved. Find those examples in your own life and you'll see you really *can* change any trait you want with the right motivation and effort, including your health.

Develop Routines

You may think of routines as boring and unimaginative, but when you're trying to change or establish a new habit, creating a routine can make it stick much faster. This tip plays on the habit research of *New York Times* reporter Charles Duhigg, who writes in *The Power of Habit* that every habit starts with a cue. That cue (like the time of day, who you're with, or the immediately preceding action) is like a subconscious kick in the pants, automatically moving us toward your routine (the habitual behavior that brings reward).

- It's 9 p.m.; time to prowl through the pantry for something sweet.

- When I meet my best friend for coffee, I always eat the scones.

- Just left my mom's, and I am *so* opening a bottle of wine when I get home.

That last one is a totally hypothetical example, Mom.

Your reset should have helped you identify some of the cues for your less-healthy routines. As an example, let's take the cues I just mentioned: In the absence of the less-healthy foods and drinks that made up your habits, you were forced to recognize the behavior ("I'm about to reach for junk food"), identify your cue ("This is a nighttime habit"; "I feel like poor food choices don't count if my friend and I both participate"; "My mom really stresses me out"), and change your behaviors in those situations.

Now you're going to turn this association around and make it work *for* you by creating a cue for the good habits you want to reinforce.

You don't need to put your whole life on autopilot to take advantage of this trick; only create specific routines around specific behaviors you want to support. Choose a few situations in which you feel your willpower getting shaky or times of day when having a routine would help you feel self-confident and in control. Then create a cue to drive you toward healthy behaviors.

One example is the common practice of getting home from work and immediately snacking, even if you're not hungry. In this case, the cue is the immediately preceding action (arriving at home), so design a new routine to follow that cue, to prevent you from ruining dinner with less-healthy foods. Your new routine could be changing into walking or exercise clothes to remind yourself that you're a healthy person with healthy habits.* (Bonus: Actually go for a short walk after dinner!) Or you could brew a cup of herbal tea every day when you get home, a soothing ritual that allows you to shift from "work mode" to "home mode." Whatever you plan, just think about using the cue to your advantage, encouraging the key in your door to trigger a healthy routine instead of the old snacking one.

Another good place to focus is your pre-bed routine. It's common to crave something sweet, salty, and crunchy before bed, often out of habit, boredom, or insomnia. A really easy cue to signify that eating time is over is brushing your teeth every night after dinner, but before your cravings start to stir. The

---

* This is a favorite trick of mine. I'm way less likely to skip the gym or raid the pantry if I'm in fitness clothing. Just the act of putting on my tights and sneakers makes me feel stronger and healthier. That's my excuse for basically living in yoga pants while writing this book.

act sends a signal to your brain that bedtime is coming, and the minty flavor reminds you that you've finished eating. In this case, you're *adding* a cue to trigger a new routine—brushing teeth after dinner, to prompt you to start winding down for bed instead of prowl through the pantry.

MORNING ROUTINE

While experts don't agree on one ideal morning routine, they do agree that employing one leads to increased willpower, more productivity, and even better health. Waking up to a routine makes you feel like you're running the day, instead of the day running you over. It helps you feel proactive instead of reactive, and ensures that you have time for your most important priorities. Over the years, I've learned that when I exercise before I start work, I'm far less likely to stress-eat, get anxious, or work too much. So I've built my morning around that healthy habit, and I follow this routine as often as possible, even when traveling. As you continue in your "healthy person" growth mind-set, think about what kind of morning routine you could build to support that notion. Perhaps you wake up and meditate, exercise, or go for a short walk; cook a healthy breakfast; write in your journal; or food prep for the day—all behaviors that will support your new healthy habits. The key is creating a routine that works for you, and then sticking to it every day until it feels effortless.

Exactly *what* you do is less important than doing something consistently. You want these routines to become habit, which reaffirms your growth mind-set, creates the cue for better habits, and frees up space in your willpower center for unexpected temptations.

Speaking of which . . .

Boost Your Willpower

When you think of "willpower," what's the scenario that comes to mind? It's probably passing on dessert after dinner or walking right past the candy dish at the office. But willpower involves a lot more than food—and understanding what willpower is and how it works can go a long way toward and keeping yourself on a healthy path.

Willpower is the ability to delay immediate gratification for the sake of long-term goals. Think of it as self-regulation or, more simply, resisting temptation. Our brains want to take the path of least resistance to whatever reward is lurking right around the corner. It's easier to sit on the couch watching *Game of Thrones* than it is to clean the kitchen. It's tastier to eat the cookies now and worry about your diet later. It feels better to snap at your colleague for taking credit for your idea, rather than biting your tongue and waiting for the right time to broach the subject.

Turning off the TV, passing on the cookie, and holding your tongue are all forms of self-regulation. In fact, any time you resist temptation or immediate gratification (like in each of the following scenarios), you are exerting willpower.

- **Not hitting snooze when your alarm goes off**
- **Committing to the gym instead of sleeping in**
- **Ignoring those seventeen Facebook notifications while you pack your work bag**
- **Drinking one cup of coffee instead of the two you really want**
- **Making scrambled eggs for breakfast instead of grabbing a muffin**
- **Not checking e-mail while driving**
- **Warming up for ten minutes instead of jumping right into your workout**
- **Not taking a selfie even though the gym lighting is excellent**
- **Not stopping for another coffee on the way to the office**
- **Not reaching for your phone at every. Single. Red. Light.**
- **Feigning interest in your boss's baby photos in the elevator**
- **Filling up your water and ignoring the donuts on the break room counter.**

And it's not even 8 a.m.

CHANGE YOUR DIET: CHECK

Poor diet and lifestyle choices are *no bueno* when it comes to willpower. Overconsuming calorie-dense, carbohydrate-dense, nutrient-poor processed foods (especially at night) leads to changes in blood sugar regulation and hormonal balance and promotes inflammation, all of which stress the body. The resulting sleep disturbances and chronic stress promote further disruptions to the brain's reward and self-regulation centers. All these factors lead to more cravings for sugar and processed carbs—which, under these circumstances, require huge amounts of willpower to resist . . . and the cycle continues. Happily, we can now check this risk factor off your list, thanks to your healthy reset diet and new food freedom habits.

Researchers agree that your willpower "bank" (the amount of energy available in the brain to exercise self-regulation and resist temptation) is a limited resource—like having $100 in a bank account. Each time you exert willpower, you withdraw a dollar—or a few. When the account is down to $0, well . . . you know the kind of decisions you make then.

The problem is that in today's world, you're constantly bombarded with temptation and the promise of reward. If you start spending your willpower dollars before you're even out the door, what do you think your balance will be by the time you get home from a tough day at the office? It's no wonder you struggle with making good choices (like resisting the lure of the pantry) late at night.

There is good news, however. By applying some smart strategies, you can actually make your willpower bank more robust and make those dollars go further than they used to.

THE NIGHT BEFORE

Improving your willpower for any given day starts the night before. Take as many decisions out of tomorrow as possible—especially the ones involving food. Lay out your clothes; prep your coffee, breakfast, and lunch; pre-pack your work bag. Try to predict ahead of time whether you'll be feeling rested enough to hit the gym, or whether you will need the extra hour of sleep. This way, your brain won't be forced to make trivial decisions early in the morning, and you'll have more willpower bucks to spend later in the day.

Also, get your butt into bed earlier.

Sleep makes ample deposits into your willpower bank, while fatigue creates stress, which compromises willpower. According to researchers, sleep is the most important step toward keeping your willpower bank full. At first, turning the TV off or putting your smartphone away by 9 p.m. may feel like a Herculean effort, but you'll more than make up for it in the morning by not having to wrestle with the snooze button. (Bonus: Eliminating the light from your phone, tablet, or television screen before bed will help you sleep better, too—the blue-wavelength light they emanate is especially disruptive to your circadian rhythm.*)

Finally, use the end of your day to make a plan for handling stressful, tempting, or unknown situations that may arise tomorrow. Some will be obvious, like a researching the menu for your business lunch so you know what you'll order, or stashing a hearty, healthy snack in your bag just in case you find yourself stuck at the office late (and hungry). Others may be more unknown, like saying to yourself, "Tomorrow is Friday. What will I do if I'm invited out for drinks after work?" Make a plan for staying true to your health commitments if you accept, or make other plans after work (like a yoga class) that are better suited to your goals.

Why go through this extra step? Because the brain loves a plan, and unfinished business tends to ping-pong around up there, creating distractions and anxiety. If you know you've got a stressful situation coming up, you may subconsciously worry about how you'll handle it—"Will I stay strong, or will I give in?" This can disrupt sleep and fire up your brain's "fear and worry" center, creating more stress and depleting willpower even further.

Welcome to the "if/then" plan.

This perhaps the most powerful tool in your food freedom toolbox. Creating an "if/then" plan for stressful or worrisome situations puts your brain at ease while helping you preserve precious willpower. The "if/then" framework is designed to identify a trigger (the "if") and employ a predetermined routine you've designed (the "then"). Research finds this structure helps you feel more in control of difficult situations, triggering a more automatic response (the activation of your healthy plan), and making you two to three times more likely to achieve your goal. Some examples:

---

* Many smartphones now have apps or settings that shift the blue light emanating from the phone screen to a less disruptive rose hue, but the jury is out on how effective these are for actually improving your sleep cycle.

- IF my business meeting runs late, THEN I'll eat the healthy emergency food stashed in my desk.

- IF I'm at happy hour and don't want a drink, THEN I'll order a sparkling water with lime, say "Not tonight, thanks" if offered, and change the subject.

- IF there's nothing I want to eat at the birthday party, THEN I'll munch on the appetizer I brought and eat a full meal when I get home.

It's also helpful to create a generic "if/then" for unknown temptations, just to reinforce the strategies you've been learning: "IF I get into a situation where I feel too pressured or tempted to make a smart choice, THEN I'll implement a ten-minute waiting period."

Finally, write your plans down. This forces you to make them clear and detailed; and the more detailed the plan, the better the chance you'll actually follow it when the situation arises. You can even go back at the end of the day and rate your plan's success on a scale of 1 (not at all successful) to 5 (knocked it out of the park) and make suggestions for improvement, so the next time that situation comes up, you'll be even better prepared to handle it.

DURING THE DAY

The best way to conserve willpower is to avoid temptation.

Duh.

Well, I know it *sounds* obvious, but if I was tough-loving you, I'd say you probably don't employ it as often as you could. The best way to start is to find areas in your life where temptations lurk, and see how many you can eliminate *before* they become a drain on your willpower.

It's time to talk about your phone.

Technology has a vampiresque impact on willpower, sucking the life out of our capacity to just say no to temptation. Research shows that resisting the lure of technology—the "ping" of an e-mail notification, the text message alert on your iPhone, all those shows you have lined up on Netflix—are especially taxing on your willpower reserve. Think about how many apps you have on your smartphone, all the various methods friends can use to connect with you, and how many times you've used technology to procrastinate. It seems pretty clear that one of the smartest moves you can make is to reduce the sheer volume of temptations that come from your beloved Internet-connected devices. I know you don't *want* to, but ask yourself this question (and do it in Siri's voice, if that helps): "What if being less obsessed with my phone helped me stay in control with my food choices, maintain a healthy waistline, and build my self-confidence?"

You're taking too long to answer. Regardless, you really should do this.

Your first mission: Turn off notifications on your smartphone and computer. The result: No more pop-up when someone hearts your Instagram photo, and no more message indicator on your e-mail icon (that triple-digit number was stressing you out, anyway), no more alerts when someone posts a new story on Snapchat. I'm not a doctor, but I'm pretty sure nobody ever died from FOMO (Fear Of Missing Out). Remove these cues, and you'll cut way down on the RIGHT THIS MINUTE WHAT IF I'M MISSING SOMETHING mentality. In addition, move your most-frequented social media apps off your home screen, so every time you make a business call or consult your calendar, you're not reminded that you haven't checked Twitter in four whole minutes.

FACEBOOK, I JUST CAN'T QUIT YOU

Why is the buzz of a new text, e-mail, or social media notification so darn addictive? Dopamine, that's why. The same neurotransmitter responsible for "wanting" and "seeking" rewarding food also really loves the promise of a new notification. Your brain associates that little ping with validation ("Someone liked my comment!"), belonging ("I'm part of this social connection!"), and seeking (discovering new music, articles, or photos of dogs who are stuck in things but doing just fine*). Sharing stuff with your social group—and netting a ton of Likes in return—feels really good, encouraging you to seek more content, to share with more people, and generate more instantaneous feedback, which feels even better . . . Given how fast the rewards pile up thanks to technology, you can get stuck in an endless loop of wanting → reward → wanting more → more reward. Plus, there's the ever-present cue: that little *chirp* or notification that precipitates you picking up your phone. No wonder it's so hard to ignore.

You should Google this. It's a thing, and it's magnificent.

Bonus: Removing notifications means you're more likely to stay on task while at work or at home, reducing the time you spend multitasking—a practice that also saps your willpower. Win-win.

Your phone isn't the only area where temptation lurks. Netflix had you hooked when it began automatically showing you the next episode in the series—it's an involuntary "opt-in" requiring *effort* to stop watching. This makes it all too likely that you'll put off meal prep, housework, or a sane bedtime routine in favor of "just one more" episode of *Orange Is the New Black*. And iTunes now sends you a love note when a new episode of your favorite show is available, which means that checking your e-mail one last time before bed may translate to 43 minutes less sleep.

If you find yourself too spent by the end of the day to resist the lure of television, try creating some rules around that, too. Set a deadline for movies (must start by 7:30 p.m., no later), institute "No TV" nights, put a limit on the number of hours you watch in any given evening, or create a rule that you don't sit down to watch TV until specific tasks have been accomplished.

One last proposed rule: No televisions, tablets, or phones in your bedroom. You hate that, but willpower really needs you to sleep, and right before bed is when you're most likely to make poor choices.

It's midnight. You can share that video of the screaming marmot tomorrow.

Now that we've covered technology, you can also make some changes to your daily routine to protect you from food-related temptation. If your co-worker's candy dish catcalls you every time you walk by, try a different route to the bathroom, and hold meetings in your cubicle, not hers. If you know your office birthday party is at 2 p.m. (and that store-bought cake won't be worth it), eat your healthy lunch right before so you show up full and satisfied. Tell your family to move their junk food to a special out-of-the-way cabinet, ask the waiter not to bring the dessert menu, and for the love of Oprah, don't go to the grocery store hungry.

Or anxious.

Or sad.

Or without a list.

Think about every possible situation in which you could simply skip the temptation instead of having to resist it, and then put a plan in place to do just that. As the old military adage says, the best defense is a good offense.

POSITIVE THINKING.

Research shows that people who (a) think positively, (b) believe willpower can be "strengthened" (there's that growth mind-set again), and (c) are generally upbeat can stretch their willpower capacity, especially early in the day. I know, easier said than done, especially on a Monday. Still, you may be surprised at how small shifts in your thinking can lead to huge improvements in your outlook. Try adding a gratitude practice to your morning routine; recognizing negative thoughts or a fixed mind-set and substituting positive ones; reading more about positive thinking to reinforce the concept; or learning how to accept "what is" and reject negative thoughts by practicing what self-help and empowerment expert Byron Katie calls The Work.*

*The Work is a simple yet powerful process of inquiry that teaches you to identify and question the thoughts that are at the root of your suffering. It's a way to understand what's hurting you, and to address the cause of your problems with clarity. For more information, see Loving What Is, by Byron Katie, or visit thework.com.

More on Willpower ...

Preparing the night before, kicking your phone out of bed, thinking happy thoughts ... we've covered a lot of territory here, but there are a few more willpower-strengthening techniques to add to your toolbox.

Another proven willpower boost (not to mention growth mind-set reinforcer, waistline buddy, and generally healthy practice) is exercise. Moving your body leads to changes in the brain that support self-control; perhaps through modulating stress, which you'll read more about in the next section.

Two key points when it comes to exercise and willpower: First, you don't have to exercise seven days a week to see the benefits. In one study, participants were asked to exercise just once a week for the first month, and three times a week for the second. After just two months, all participants demonstrated significant improvement in self-regulation and emotional control, as well as a decrease in stress. That's a pretty good return on investment. Second, you don't have to exercise at high intensity for this to work—walking, yoga, weightlifting, a dance class, or playing soccer with your kids all do the trick.

In addition, adding a meditation practice to your day can help with self-regulation, stress management, and even balancing hormone levels. (In fact, the more research I do, the more I'm convinced meditation makes *everything* better.) You needn't sit in lotus position for hours on end; studies show that just eight weeks of brief daily training (about a half hour a day) can boost self-regulation, and comments from the study suggest that even ten minutes a day could be beneficial.

A basic routine looks like this:

- Choose a time of day that will allow you to be consistent in your efforts. Adding meditation to your morning routine is a great way to start the day off calm and centered, but you can meditate any time.

- Choose a quiet place where you won't be disturbed.

- Get into a comfortable seated position, using blocks, bolsters, pillows, and any other props that work for you. (Don't lie down— you're not relaxing into sleep!)

- Set a gentle alarm for a time that feels reasonable for you. Start with just five to ten minutes if you're new to the practice.

- Now just sit. You can focus on your breath, counting while you inhale and exhale; practice a mantra (the Hindu *Om*, a motivational mantra like "Change my thoughts, change the world," or a loving kindness mantra like "May I be happy. May I be well. May I be safe. May I be peaceful and at ease."); or visualize breathing in light and breathing out stress.

- When you find yourself distracted, simply return to your chosen focus. This will happen approximately 173 times in ten minutes, but that's actually a good thing; the act of gently shifting your brain back to your focus is part of the process. That's why meditation is called a *practice*.

- When your time is up, gently return to your body and your surroundings, wiggling your fingers and toes, slowly opening your eyes, and standing.

If you'd rather be more directed in your practice, there are many smart-phone apps (like Headspace or Calm) to guide you through meditation. The website Zen Habits has a great tutorial to get you started (zenhabits.net/meditation), and the book *10% Happier* by Dan Harris offers some very practical tips for establishing a meditation practice in a highly entertaining, often irreverent fashion, which may appeal more to all of your type-A, high-energy, can't-sit-still rebels.

Not that I'd know anything about that.

ONE MOMENT MEDITATION

You can even train yourself to use "one-moment meditation" to help get you through a tough situation. One study found that practicing mindfulness in the moment is a quick and efficient strategy to foster self-control, even when you're feeling like all willpower has abandoned you. Psychotherapist Martin Boroson has developed an easy tutorial for practicing mindfulness in the moment; visit his website at onemomentmeditation.com.

Finally, as I alluded to earlier, adopt a growth mind-set here, too—then create a situation to prove you're actually better at implementing self-control. Choose to believe (as most research suggests) that willpower works like a muscle; you can strengthen it by working it. You can do this by picking a low-risk task (flossing, doing all the dishes after dinner, or writing in your journal) and committing to it for 30 days. Consistently resist the temptation to bail on your task, and you'll gain willpower strength over time.

Manage Stress

Finally, the big-picture tip that probably could have gone first because it's that important: Reduce your stress. (Aside: It's featured last because if you do all the other stuff that comes before it, this one is going to be way easier.)

You don't need a Genius Bar appointment to know that chronic stress ruins everything. It promotes anxiety, heart disease, weight gain, depression, sleep disturbances, impaired concentration, neurological disorders, immune dysfunction, chronic pain, cravings, and bad hair days. Okay, not that last one ... but maybe, because when you're under chronic stress, *everything* looks harder, feels worse, and provokes more worry than it should.

Most people think of stress in terms of hating their job, worrying about money, or feeling out of control. That last one is closest to the truth; stress is defined as a perceived threat to your physical or social safety. The "chronic" part just means it's ongoing or prolonged, instead of acute (short term). Need an example?

Acute stress is being chased by a snarling dog from the mailbox back to your house. It's *really* scary, but it's over quickly—as soon as you slam your front door, you know you're safe and can relax and recover from the experience. Chronic stress is being chased by a snarling dog all day long, everywhere you go. You wake up, the dog is there, so you start running. You get out of a meeting, and there's the dog, so you start running again. You lie down at night and you can still hear him breathing, just waiting for you to get up again so he can chase you some more.

That's not normal.

In the prehistoric world, stressors were intense but brief: you were chased by a boar, fell down an embankment into the river, or were confronted by a rival intent on stealing your wild game. In today's world, however, stressors are much different: a perpetually packed schedule; a 60-hour-a-week job; balancing responsibilities as a spouse, parent, employee, and friend; pressures to "keep up" with the neighbors and achieve your own goals.

Your stress-response system was not designed to be constantly activated, yet this is what most people deal with, day in and day out. We are on perpetual high alert, because our brain interprets the constant stress of life as it would the stress of constantly being chased. That's the first truth about stress: Perception is reality, so when you think a stressful thought, your body responds as if something stressful is actually happening. The second truth: Your body responds the same way to psychological stress as it does to physical stress. That means hating your job and being chased by a snarling dog are basically the same thing. The third truth about stress: There are more stress inputs in today's modern world than ever, and you probably didn't even recognize all the ones affecting you until now.

This is very depressing. Which is stressful. I'M SORRY. Please keep reading.

In the wild, where stressors are intense but brief, your body has an elegant and balanced way of coping. Let's say you really are being chased by that barking dog. At the first signs of stress, chemical messengers prepare your body to fight or flee. Blood sugar is released from temporary storage sites into the bloodstream for immediate energy; the immune system activates in case you get hurt; and digestion shuts down, because who has time to break down a steak when you're running for your life? Once you're safe inside your house, other messengers bring all those systems back to a healthy balance: Blood sugar returns to your muscles, the immune system calms down, and digestion comes back online, which brings your body back into homeostasis. See? Not all stress is bad! It helps your body adapt, get stronger, and survive, if presented in the right context and dose.

SOURCES OF STRESS

n today's busy, modern world, stress comes from a variety of sources, both physical and psychological. From this still-not-exhaustive list, you'll probably recognize more than one cause of stress in your own life. An even bigger bummer: They all add up, compounding the havoc stress wreaks on your body and brain.

PHYSICAL SOURCES: Manual labor, hard training, illness, infections, injury, surgery, pain, disability, malnutrition/undereating, sleep deprivation, inflammation, toxic exposure, allergies, food sensitivities

PSYCHOLOGICAL SOURCES: Anger, fear, worry, anxiety, depression, guilt, shame, abandonment, rejection, betrayal, jealousy, comparison, social isolation, divorce, death, physical/sexual/emotional abuse, financial, career, relationships, children, self-worth, self-esteem

In today's world, though, where stressors are intense *and* ongoing, the stress response is overdone. The brain constantly perceives stress, so the stress response is constantly activated. It's like you're encountering that snarling dog 17 times a day, and some encounters last three hours. This jacks up all kinds of stuff in your body.

Chronic activation of the stress response changes neurotransmitters like dopamine, oxytocin, and serotonin, as well as feel-good opioids, making you "want" high-reward things (like chocolate) more, but "like" them less. You've probably already experienced this; you imagine a treat, how good it will taste, and how much better it will make you feel, but once you actually eat it . . . meh. The anticipation was huge, but you didn't enjoy it nearly as much as you imagined you would. (Oh, but you ate it all anyway, because the "want" is hard to resist.)

Chronic stress also affects blood sugar regulation and hormones like insulin, so your cells aren't as good at managing energy. This leaves you with blood sugar dips that feel a lot like hunger, and signals your brain that you need fast energy in the form of sugar—NOW. Stress also specifically targets your brain's prefrontal cortex, the home of executive function and self-regulation (also known as willpower). These three issues join together to form the perfect sugar-storm: Under chronic stress, you want rewarding foods more but enjoy them less when you actually eat them. Your body isn't as good at managing blood sugar, making you hungry even though you've eaten plenty of calories. Your brain sucks at converting sugar into energy, which makes it think you just need more sugar to function. And amid all this, your willpower center is just phoning it in.

What does this have to do with maintaining your food freedom? If you get one thing from this section, get this:

Stress makes you crave . . .

And not grilled chicken and steamed broccoli, either. Under stress, your body demands the sugary, processed, carb-dense, rewarding stuff. And because it's biological—an automatic response to a perceived threat—no amount of willpower can completely combat these cravings. To retain your food freedom, successfully manage cravings, and stay in control, the most important thing you can do is manage your stressors. All of them.

And no, I'm not going to tell you to "just relax," because never in the history of relaxing has anyone ever relaxed by being told to just relax.

Control the Things You Can Control

Here's how:

SLEEP: Go to bed earlier, sleep later when you can, and create a healthy nighttime routine; no screens an hour before bed! If you live in a brightly lit area, customize your bedroom with blackout curtains, and remove all electronic lights from your sleeping environment, including LED alarm clocks, iPads, laptops, and nightlights. Studies also show you'll sleep better if your bedroom is cool, so turn your thermostat way down at night—and be prepared for a rather brisk a.m. potty trip. Bonus: Being overtired hits your prefrontal cortex especially hard, so using these tips to restore good sleep will also reboot your willpower.

EXERCISE: Modulate your intensity, frequency, or duration. (My rule of thumb: You can go hard, you can go often, you can go long. Pick two.) In times of stress, reduce the intensity first—try long, slow distance exercise in nature, like hikes, easy bike rides, or walks. These are healthy for the immune system without being stressful on the body.

ENVIRONMENT: Get outside! Studies show even small amounts of time spent in "green spaces," like a park, your backyard, or the woods, moderates stress. Add a short walk to your lunch routine, eat breakfast outside on the patio, and in warmer months, bare your body for regular, safe sun exposure while you're out there to soak up that vitamin D.

SOCIAL: Connect with real people. No, not via text message. In-person social connection is a powerful stress-reducer, so reach out to friends, family, or a trusted counselor. Volunteer work can also be profoundly stress-reducing, even if giving away some of your already limited time sounds counterintuitive. For bonus points, combine healthy exercise and green spaces with your social connections: invite a friend for a walk in the park or a hike in the mountains.

PSYCHOLOGICAL: Reconnect with your faith, seek the counsel of a mentor or pastor, or explore different therapeutic modalities, like energy healing, massage, or acupuncture. Improve how you respond to difficult people or situations using techniques like Byron Katie's The Work (see page 115). Build quiet time into your morning routine, to start the day off calmly.

E.R.C.: Finally, when stress feels overwhelming and you don't know where to start, think Eliminate, Reduce, and Cope. Make a list of your stressors, first identifying those you can *eliminate* completely. Cancel the social obligations that feel the most burdensome, politely decline the offer to join the Parent-Teacher Association, and tell your in-laws it's just not a good time for a visit. Then figure out which stressors you can *reduce*. Let the house stay a little messier than you'd like, take a break from tension-filled interactions with your co-worker, and put a freeze on nonessential purchases for the month. Finally, identify those stressors with which you must simply *cope*. A newborn baby is something you just have to work around, so create strategies to help you manage the sleep deprivation and routine disruption for the next few months, using the tools you've learned here.

MAGNESIUM SUPPLEMENTS

Smart supplementation can also support your everyday stress-reducing practices. Stress at the cellular level drives down magnesium levels, which makes it hard to relax (especially at bedtime) and harder for your body to utilize glucose as energy. You can take a patented magnesium form called Magtein (like that offered by NOW Foods), which is designed to cross the blood-brain barrier more effectively, or supplement with a powdered magnesium citrate like Natural Calm. Split your dose up throughout the day, taking some midday and the rest just before bed. If sleep is your biggest issue, try an all-natural supplement like Dr. Kirk Parsley's Sleep Remedy (docparsley.com), which contains magnesium and other micronutrients designed to promote deep, natural sleep.

Happier Ever After

After reading this chapter, you'll have a lot of tools in your food freedom toolbox; enough to help you MacGyver your way out of some of the stickiest food situations. In addition to those in-the-moment techniques designed to help you manage cravings, evaluate your options, and retain willpower, you now have four big-picture strategies to support your new, healthy lifestyle:

- Adopt a growth mind-set

- Develop routines

- Boost willpower

- Manage stress

Ideally, with these tools (along with ample opportunities to practice), you'll be able to maintain your food freedom indefinitely; indulging when it's worth it, declining when it isn't, and feeling satisfied and in control.

Full disclosure: That's probably not going to happen just yet. Your food freedom journey is still new, and old habits die hard. At some point in the months following your reset, 90 percent of you will find yourself on a slippery slide back to Old Behaviorsville, waking up one morning realizing you aren't as energetic, happy, or confident as you used to be.

Also, someone shrunk your jeans, which is sneaky and mean.

In the past, this would have been met with shock and confusion. You were doing SO WELL. You were feeling SO GOOD. How could you have let this happen?

Well I'm telling you now so you're not surprised... *something* happened, and chances are, it's one of the five scenarios I'm about to outline in chapter 9. So let's target them now, to prevent the situation from happening in the first place, control it while it's happening, or at the very least, recover from it more gracefully than falling face first into a pint of ice cream.

ACKNOWLEDGE WHEN YOU'RE STARTING TO SLIP

SPOT YOUR TRIGGERS

Your Food Freedom car will, at some point, meander off the road and slowly roll—or plunge headfirst—into a ravine of comfort foods: chocolate, donuts (chocolate donuts), ice cream, chips, bread, wine, cheese. This is likely to happen even if your reset was insanely successful, and you emerged like a food freedom phoenix from the ~~crumbs~~ ashes. Why? Because changing your habits is hard, you're still new at this, and you haven't completely established healthy habits in place of all the old ones.

It turns out habits aren't something you can erase; you can only overwrite them with different ones. This means old habits really do die hard; something you may have noticed if the following situation has ever happened to you:

You've been driving the same way to work every day for years. Then you relocate to a new home or apartment in a different part of town. You create a new route to and from work, and if you're like most people, you drive the exact same way every day. You do this for weeks and weeks, until one evening when you're stressed and distracted after a long day, you find yourself taking the wrong exit—the one heading toward your old house.

Awareness is hard to maintain 24/7, especially with something as habitual as driving.

Or eating.

In many cases, your most familiar (and detrimental) eating habits have become as automatic as driving. You don't think about getting home from work, cracking a bottle of wine, and snacking on some cheese and crackers; it's just what you do. It's automatic to reach for a soda or chocolate at 3 p.m. to stay alert, say "It's go time" when arriving at a party, or dig into the ice cream every time you're home alone.

Overwriting these ingrained habits requires constant awareness, consistency in your approach, and practicing the new habits day in and day out. And that's *really* hard when it comes to eating, something we do multiple times a day. People have strong emotional attachments to food, and it provides incredible reward. Compounding the situation, when you're under stress, without a plan, and/or experiencing a negative emotion, the brain is far more likely to revert back to what is familiar and rewarding.

You attend birthday parties. You go on vacation. There's a holiday. Your significant other dumps you. You get sad. You get anxious. You get bored. You get sick. Your mom visits. You have a business lunch. Your plane is delayed. Life constantly throws curve balls at your day-to-day routine, and unless you have a solid strategy for maintaining the healthy eating plan that's right for you, any one of these scenarios could knock you right off your food freedom path.

This is why your Food Freedom plan specifically accounts for losing control of your new, healthy habits and slipping back into old ones. I wish I could promise that your reset will be so effective it will totally overwrite all your bad habits; that it will rehabilitate your emotional relationship with food so effectively that you'll let go of all past associations and will never again find yourself unconsciously taking your "old exit."

That would be lovely, but it's not realistic.

Without a frank acknowledgment of what's far more likely to happen, you'll be caught off guard, without a plan and stressed about it. Which only cues the brain to return to old, familiar, comforting habits—the exact thing you're desperately trying to prevent. Which brings us to the tough-love Step 3 of the Food Freedom plan.

STEP 3:
ACKNOWLEDGE WHEN YOU'RE STARTING TO SLIP.

- Watch out for the "slow slide"
- Beware of common triggers
- Commit to honesty and self-awareness

You're probably already aware of a few situations that can easily derail your commitment to healthy eating (I'm looking at you, Thanksgiving through New Year's). From my own personal and professional experience, I've pinpointed five common triggers that are itching to unravel your food freedom gains. Let's identify each one, and create a plan for how to handle it.

Trigger #1: The Slow Slide

The most common descent back into old habits is the slow slide: a gradual decline in awareness and a laziness in exercising your "worth it" muscles. It progresses so slowly that you're not even aware it's happening, until one morning you wake up and think, "Whoa, my energy is dragging, my Sugar Dragon is raging, my skin is breaking out, and I can't button my pants. What happened?"

Here is a cold, hard truth:

This will happen to you.

At some point after your reset is over (much sooner for some people than others), you will find yourself at least partially entrenched in your old habits, perhaps without much of a grasp on how you ended up there.

Here's what happened: It's really difficult to maintain so much awareness about off-plan food choices, especially if the practice of doing so is new. It can be physically and emotionally demanding. Over time, you'll find yourself saying, "Close enough" more often than asking yourself, "Wait, is this really worth it?" You'll feel like you've been so good, you can afford to relax for a little while. You'll start grandfathering in worth-it choices; once you've accepted a food as worth it once, you'll just leave it in your daily diet, despite the fact that if you reanalyzed it critically, you'd realize it wasn't *always* worth it.

Sweetened coffee creamers do this to me. On a whim, I'll buy the vanilla coconut milk version and add it to my decaf one morning. It's a delicious treat, so the next morning I'll want it again, and the next, and the next . . . Eventually I realize my creamer consumption has switched over to automatic, which is leading me to drink more coffee than usual and forcing me to fight off new sugar cravings during the day.

No matter how vigilant you are, in the beginning it's hard to resist the slow slide. You've got just a month or two of food freedom competing with decades of old habits and rewarding foods. So don't beat yourself up about it, or avoid dealing with it by pretending it's not happening. The key is realizing that you're starting down the slow slide before the effects mushroom out of control. Let's put some cross-checks in place to help you stay aware and prevent you from slipping too far.

A food journal is the first tool in your slow slide arsenal. You don't have to track calories or list every ingredient, but writing down your meals for a few days can help you spot areas where off-plan foods have made a quiet but steady reappearance. You may still be eating "Whole30-ish," but if your food log shows that you're having something sweet after every lunch and dinner, that should be enough to make you pause and ask, "Am I slipping back into a bad habit here?"

A journal can also help you pinpoint any "gateway drug": foods or beverages that open the door to the slow slide of poor food choices. These individual triggers are different for everyone, but if you thought about it for a few minutes, you could probably identify at least one or two that are surefire Sugar Dragon agitators for you. If you start paying attention when you indulge and log the resultant cravings or food choices in a journal, you'll be in a far better position to identify the culprits right then and there.

SAMPLE JOURNAL

Make a notation every time you choose to indulge. It doesn't have to be a dissertation; keep it short and direct:

- *Cupcake at birthday party, ate it all, no seconds.*
- *Fresh bread at the restaurant, ate three slices mindlessly, ordered cake for dessert, wasn't that good but ate it anyway.*

Create a "control scale" of 1 to 5, with 1 being supremely in control (Sugar Dragon is a tame gecko) and 5 is totally out of control (Sugar Dragon razed a whole village). Also keep in mind that your trigger may not be a usual suspect, like chocolate or wine. For Julie K. of Michigan, diet soda is a gateway beverage. She says, "When my reset is over, if I go back to the soda, all the other bad stuff follows. If I just stay off it, then mentally I am still on my healthy eating program and everything else falls into place." Others cite salty food as a trigger, wanting something sweet immediately afterward to balance the flavors. A few Whole30ers even mentioned cheese as a trigger food. It doesn't matter if your triggers are textbook or seem strange to you—the point is to spot them, because a hidden trigger is a lot easier to pull.

Once you identify those foods that will send you off the rails, tread carefully. Decide ahead of time how much you'll eat, and create a rule that you'll stop with just that treat. Portion out a serving that will feel satisfying to you instead of eating directly from the bag or box. Eat consciously, even more slowly than usual. And do I really have to caution you against combining these foods with alcohol?

You could also choose not to eat them at all.

I have a friend who is infamous for how fast he can take down a jar of sunflower seed butter. After his first Whole30 (during which he ate none, recognizing it as a habit he wanted to break), he reintroduced it to his pantry . . . and quickly realized that, for him, there are no brakes on this particular food. He likes it, sure, but having it on hand just stresses him out, because he's always afraid he'll come home one night too tired, hungry, or emotional to resist. So, he stopped buying it. There are other delicious healthy fats, and for him, removing just this one item was the key to staying in control with the rest of his diet.

If you make sunflower seed butter, you're bummed, because he was a really good customer, but from a food freedom perspective, that's a very smart move.

You can also tackle the slow slide by taking daily or weekly stock of how you're feeling, and compare it to how you felt after your reset. How easily your pants are buttoning is another pretty good (but not foolproof) indication of how things are going. It could be a sign that you've been indulging a little more often than you've realized and have put on some weight as a result. It could also mean you've been exercising and putting on muscle mass, retaining water thanks to your monthly cycle, or maybe your wife really did throw your jeans in the dryer on high. Use how your clothes fit as a general trend, but don't make it your only barometer. For other physical signs, look to your skin (still clear?), joints (are they swollen; do your rings still fit?), or belly bloat (are you consistently puffy?) to help you see the physical effects of a slow slide.

GET TECHY

Wear a fitness tracker? Your wearable device can also alert you to subtle signs of a slow slide. Using your device, monitor steps taken and how long and well you're sleeping. If you notice a trend (you're sleeping worse, hitting snooze more often, or losing motivation to hit the gym or go for a walk), it's time to do a thorough evaluation of your diet and see if a slow slide is to blame.

Sometimes, the fix is easy. In my case, I just stop using any and all creamer and return to drinking my coffee black; my cravings disappear, and all is well. If there's just one item in your rotation that seems to always throw you off track, like Julie's diet soda, my friend's sunflower seed butter, or maybe something else (*hello*, WINE), you can probably just cut out that one item for a while, get back on track, then if you choose to, commit to reintroducing it slowly and deliberately, paying better attention this time.

Finally, if you've got a few different contributors, create some short-term rules to help get yourself back on track, targeting the suspected culprits. (Common offenders include sugar, alcohol, chocolate, crunchy salty things, and baked goods. Lentils are rarely a gateway food.) You can think of these rules like a mini reset, designed to provide you with enough structure to see it through while still giving you the flexibility to make your own decisions. Guidelines like, "No desserts for a week," "No more chips while watching movies," or "No more baked goods at breakfast" may be just the push you need to stop your slow slide and get back to feeling awesome.

Trigger #2: Vacations

Vacations practically guarantee that your normal healthy routine will self-eject out the window, especially if you're traveling to an exotic location known for its delicious cuisine. (Disneyland does not count.) These special trips offer the opportunity to sample foods and beverages you've always wanted to try: pasta in Italy, tacos in Mexico, naan in India, or champagne in France. Since you're only there for a short visit and likely won't be returning anytime soon, food freedom will encourage you to explore, savor, and indulge to your heart's content . . . but still carefully, deliberately, and with awareness.

You're not off the hook just because you're in the birthplace of gelato.

Your new food freedom strategy is designed to avoid all the things that used to happen when you took a vacation. Allow me to paint that not-so-pretty postcard picture:

You crash-diet before your vacay to fit into your swimsuit/look good in photos/buy yourself a little caloric wiggle room, because you know you're about to pig out. Your diet ends just before vacation starts, leaving you metabolically slower, willpower depleted, and with massive "The plane's about to land" cravings. Then you hit your vacation destination, where your normal routine (work, chores, exercise, diet) don't apply, and your actions feel like they just don't count.

Because VACATION.

You give your prefrontal cortex (willpower center) the week off and proceed to eat and drink All the Things because you're on this trip, you prepared for this with your crash diet, and you already told yourself you could. You certainly don't think about what you're eating or the consequences, because who wants to think about unpleasant stuff like *consequences* on a vacation?

You return from vacation needing a vacation, feeling lethargic, bloated, cranky, and chubby. You swore when you got home, you'd get back to your healthy diet, but your body and brain are still in fiesta mode, and temptations are hard to resist . . . so your poor dietary habits continue for a few days after your vacation is over. Okay, a week. Well, maybe a month. At which point you realize you've gained 6 pounds, and you return to the crash diet.

While that sounds like an awful lot of fun (Sarcasm Threat Level: Fuchsia), that's not going to happen anymore. The good news is that now, thanks to Step 3, you have a plan to manage your vacation in a way that keeps you feeling in control, with lots of energy and a healthy body composition, while still enjoying the treats your destination has to offer.

PRE-VACATION: What you do in the days leading up to your vacation plays an important role in how gracefully you transition back to the real world upon return, so listen up:

Do not go off the rails before your trip even starts.

You know what I'm talking about . . . the whole, "Well, as of Saturday I'll be drinking wine, so I may as well have a glass when I get home from work." The thought is tempting, but do not do this. In fact, do the opposite.

Before your vacation, do not binge, but don't diet, either. Instead, try a mini reset. Get back into the groove of clean eating in the week(s) before you leave. Remind yourself how amazing it feels, how righteous it feels, to eat only foods that make you healthier. Get back to a place of good sleep, rockin' energy, and a flatter stomach. Remind your body that feeling any less good than this is kind of a bummer.

For me, this takes three days, but for someone newer to food freedom, it may take a week or two. Start early, and commit to the program right up through the moment you set foot in your vacation destination. Going into the trip feeling clean, light, fresh, and amazing will do wonders for your willpower when tempted with so much of the not-worth-it-but-it's-sitting-right-there-and-it-has-an-umbrella-in-it! drinks and foods you'll encounter on your trip.

DURING VACATION: While you're on your trip, you'll be following the same Food Freedom plan—you'll just have more opportunities to practice it. Thanks to your mini reset, it should be way easier to implement.

Continue to individually evaluate every potentially less-healthy food you're thinking about eating, asking yourself, "Is this worth it? Is this special enough? Is this delicious enough? Is it going to mess me up?" Pass on the stuff that doesn't cut the mustard (bar peanuts, local variations of the same old candy you have at home, the bread basket with hard, cold rolls), and enjoy what passes your test in the same deliberate, mindful, one-bite-at-a-time manner. Some days, you may find you stick to basically reset-friendly foods all day, because nothing was worth it. Excellent—and you didn't miss out on a thing, because according to the expert (you), there was nothing to miss. Other days, you may decide to indulge in something at every single meal. Also excellent, because you're making the choice deliberately, you're still in control, and you're not buying into the idea that just because you're on vacation, your choices have no consequences.

A margarita is still a margarita, even if you are in Cabo.

In the past, you might have found your vacation high hampered by worry over how much you were indulging, how loud your Sugar Dragon was roaring, and how much you dreaded coming back to the real world carrying all this vacation food baggage. This time, you have a plan. The minute you get home, you're going right back on a mini reset: Do not pass go. Do not collect two extra pieces of cheesecake. Do not even consider one last glass of wine the night before you go back to work.

When you think about it, it actually sounds kind of comforting, doesn't it? No matter how your vacation leaves you feeling, you have a proven, solid plan for regaining food freedom fast. It should set your mind at ease, and allow you to truly enjoy those worth-it foods you're savoring during your time away.

WHAT THE HELL?

Note: It is a decidedly unscientific fact that alcohol amplifies the "What the Hell" Effect by 178 percent. Indulge in booze carefully, or you may find yourself facedown in a pile of churros after those one (no, two . . . make that three!) poolside tequila shots.

POST-VACATION: Your post-vacation mind-set (and body-set) is going to depend on what you chose to eat and drink during your trip, and whether you let yourself slide down the slippery slope of the WTH Effect. Ideally, you return feeling almost as good as you did when you left—not heavy or bloated; digestive system intact; cravings relatively under control. Maybe even a little tan. Or the opposite: You return home feeling like a chunky, tired, sugar-driven shell of your former self.

If that is the case, I hope you had a *really* great trip.

Either way, the plane ride or drive home is the perfect time to prep yourself for what is ahead. This is going to sound familiar . . . it's time for another mini reset, for as long as it takes to start feeling happy, energetic, craving-free, and back in control. This could be a few days or a few weeks, depending on how far you went off the rails and how much you struggled to maintain conscious decision-making while on vacation. When you think you're ready to come off, deliberately add two more days. This will test whether your brain is really in a good place, or if you're subconsciously rushing the process at the behest of tenacious, clinging cravings.

If you're unreasonably annoyed at the idea of two more days, it's a good thing you added two more days.

In some instances, you may choose to add additional rules to your program. I always add the clause that I can't eat after dinner (no dessert) for the first few days after a vacation, because I always come home with strong cravings. You may decide not to snack, or not to eat too much dried fruit or nut butters, or to make sure you exercise for the first three days in a row post-vacation. Do this, plus your designated reset protocol, for as long as it takes for food freedom to feel effortless again.

REINTRODUCE . . . AGAIN!

Once your reset is over, it's time to carefully and systematically reintroduce. Yes, again! Every time you reintroduce, you learn a little more about how that particular food affects your body and brain. Don't waste the opportunity of another clean slate—reintroduce conscientiously and pay attention. You might be surprised to find that post-vacation, your definition of "worth it" in your everyday life has changed for the healthier.

Trigger #3: Holidays

Holidays are like mini vacations, where you tell yourself the consequences don't count. After all, "'Tis the season," amirite? Of course, President's Day or Veteran's Day probably don't invoke as many fond childhood food memories or present the same major opportunities for overconsumption as Thanksgiving or Christmas. In fact, some holidays won't require much (if any) strategizing, but *do* present the perfect opportunity for taking your food freedom skills out on the town.

Employing your Food Freedom plan during low-pressure holidays will let you practice your "worth it" skills and give you an important win by reinforcing the idea that holidays don't have to be nutritional free-for-alls to be celebratory. In fact, the more you shift your association of "holiday" away from "food-a-go-go" to "today we honor special people" or "a chance to connect with family and friends," the more that association will stick when the Big Three (Thanksgiving, Christmas/Hanukkah/Kwanzaa, and New Year's) roll around.

During an Independence Day celebration, grill some veggie and chicken kabobs, make a potato salad, and enjoy some fresh watermelon, then decide if a less-healthy treat (a cold beer, ice cream, or chips and salsa) may be worth it as an add-on. On Easter, cook a turkey or lamb chops with lots of veggie sides and make a green salad, then ask yourself whether you need candy eggs or marshmallow chicks to make the afternoon complete. On Valentine's Day, think about how many heart-shaped chocolates you *really* need to eat to make the evening romantic.

That might be none. Just sayin'.

Now, on to the big ones.

Most of us (turkeys not withstanding) have fond memories of Thanksgiving. Like many holidays, food takes center stage on the fourth Thursday of November, then again during ChristmaHanaKwanzika (or Festivus, if I'm being totally politically correct) and New Year's Eve. And it's not like the weeks in between are health-fests, either . . . Let's just say it's no coincidence that diet books begin flying off the shelves and gyms are packed to capacity on January 2.

Science reports that on average, you only gain about a pound during the holidays, but minor weight gain isn't the worst or only fallout—what about the bloating, lethargy, breakouts, sleep disruptions, guilt, and a fire-breathing Sugar Dragon inciting irresistible cravings long after the tinsel and lights have come down?

When it comes to the year-end holidays, you need a robust plan. The social pressures of the season, the stress they tend to bring, and the pervasiveness of less-healthy drinks, treats, and desserts make it mega-hard to resist temptation. This plan will look a lot like your plan for vacations, with a pre-Thanksgiving reset, a mid-holiday commitment to conscientious dietary off-roading, and a post–New Year's reset. You can also throw in mini resets (as short as a few days) between holidays or events, to keep you on track throughout the hustle and bustle of office parties, family reunions, and special dinners.

The holidays are also time to reconnect with family and friends, some of whom you see just once a year. Unlike your close friends and co-workers, these people may not know about the small changes you've been making every day to improve your health, so your new dietary habits may be surprising or confusing to them. This is especially true of your grandmother, who in all likelihood has spent the last few decades feeding you pasta and pastries as a way to show her love.

Walking up to the holiday table and passing on the marshmallow-brown-sugar-sweet-potato casserole for the first time in, well, EVER, may provoke questions. Now is not the time to quote *Food Freedom Forever* or give a lecture on the digestive perils of FODMAPs. And definitely don't tell your grandma that her gingerbread cookies make your Sugar Dragon roar.

Instead, employ this specific four-part game plan designed to help you preemptively manage conversations with family and friends.

STEP 1: Well before the holiday, schedule time to speak with key family members about your commitment to new healthy habits over the holiday, and share your personal reasons for wanting to stick to it. Now is not the time to quote a scientific study or come out of the gate defensively. Speak from your heart. Share your struggles with food, the success you've had with your new Food Freedom plan, and why you need to stay committed to taking care of *you* during the holidays.

If they seem annoyed or you suspect they think you're being silly, acknowledge it. Say, "I know an 'announcement' like this seems dramatic, but this is really important to me, which is why I'm sharing it with you. I'll make it super easy for you—in fact, you won't even notice I'm eating a little differently, and my holidays will be so much happier because I've made this commitment to my health."

DON'T SHARE SPECIFICS

Note: You haven't talked about the specifics of your reset or Food Freedom plan yet—just your personal reasons for wanting to stay committed to a healthy, balanced diet over the holidays. If you open this conversation with, "Hey, I won't be eating bread, milk, cheese, or dessert on Thanksgiving—just letting you know," the conversational train you were hoping to board will derail fast.

STEP 2: After you have their support, it's time to consider what they're planning to serve and how that fits in with your new healthy eating plan. Focus on the foods you *will* be eating, not all the stuff you won't be. Find the common ground for them, and all of a sudden this holiday dinner actually sounds pretty easy.

Ask about the menu, and internally evaluate what you'll be able to eat and what you'll want to pass up. (For instance, the turkey is good to go, but the gravy or stuffing will have gluten, and you're avoiding that.) Then create a plan with your family to make their dishes a good fit for you. Relatively easy requests include, "Can you set aside a plain sweet potato for me before you mash them all with cream?"; "Can you save me some steamed green beans before you mix them into the casserole?"; "Can you put the dressing for the salad on the side?" That's minimal extra work for your family and means you'll get to enjoy these nostalgic side dishes, too.

STEP 3: BYOSD (Bring Your Own Side Dish). Since you'll now have a good idea of what will be served, tell your family that you'd really like to contribute to the gathering. Phrase it like this: "I've been teaching myself to cook and came across this recipe that sounded perfect for Thanksgiving. I'd really like to make it for the family. Can we serve it with your potatoes and green beans?"

This works especially well with dessert. Bring a fruit-based, gluten-free, or dairy-free dessert that also fits your healthy eating plan, and make enough for everyone to enjoy. You can never have too many desserts at these holiday gatherings, and chances are people will appreciate having at least one lighter, healthier offering.

STEP 4: Relax, and roll with it. Come the big day, if your mother forgets and puts croutons in the salad or pours gravy on your turkey, don't make a big deal about it. Unless you have a serious sensitivity or allergy to a particular ingredient, just scrape off the gravy, or eat around the croutons—but don't use this as an excuse to "what the hell" with dinner rolls and apple pie.

Finally, take a moment during dinner to compliment the chefs and say a heartfelt thank-you to your family for supporting you in your commitment. They will appreciate hearing how grateful you are and will be far more likely to stay supportive of your new, healthy habits if you show them how much it means to you. And who knows—this experience may prompt family members to ask you more about the food freedom program and your experience.

Just don't talk about it at the table.

Now, I'd like to offer an additional reminder when it comes to special occasions like your anniversary or birthday. By following your "worth it" assessment and understanding that "it's delicious" is reason enough, you've already learned that it doesn't have to be a special occasion to indulge. Here's the flip side:

You also don't have to indulge just because it's a special occasion.

You're an adult with a car, money, and free will. You can buy a cupcake, a bottle of wine, or a cheesecake any time you want, always and forever. You don't have to wait for your birthday or a special occasion, because your true enjoyment of the experience makes it special. But if the special day rolls around and in that moment, you decide you're just as happy sticking to a healthy template and skipping all desserts or drinks, *you should do that.*

EMPLOY "IF/THEN" PLANS

Creating "if/then" plans here is also a smart move. Imagine the pushback or pressure you may feel during the holiday, and craft a plan to handle it. One effective tool: predicting the responses you may get from friends and family on the big day, either because you didn't get the chance to speak with them or because they're still convinced you can't properly celebrate without gorging on sugar.

IF...	THEN...
your mom says, *"But it's Christmas—just relax and enjoy yourself,"*	you'll respond, "I totally will, Mom! I'm just not going to fall face first into the whoopie pies this year—one will be plenty."
your sister says, *"You may be on this funny diet, but we sure aren't,"*	you'll respond, "I know—and I don't care what anyone eats today! It's not about the food, it's about spending time with all of you."
your grandmother says, *"But you always loved my chocolate-chip cookies,"*	you'll respond, "And I still do, but I'm stuffed right now. Can I bring one home so I can really enjoy it later?"

Remember, you aren't giving yourself "permission" to eat less-healthy food ahead of time. (Refer back to "cheat days" on page 99) You don't need permission, you're not a child, and you can have it any time you want. Plus, granting yourself permission ahead of time (before you even know whether or not you actually *want* it) + highly rewarding, right-there-in-front-of-you temptation = trouble on the conscious, deliberate decision-making front.

Case in point: It's your birthday, and you're going to a fancy new restaurant that's known for its elaborate $12 craft cocktails. You've already decided you will have one; after all, it's a celebration! You arrive at the restaurant, look at the drink menu, and realize nothing is really calling your name. In fact, you feel so good tonight (and have plans to hit the gym in the morning) that you'd really feel better just ordering sparkling water. But you already told yourself you can have the drink. So what happens?

You order one anyway because it's tempting, and, according to your brain, the minute you walked into that restaurant, the plane had landed. You end up drinking something you're not really in love with, knowing deep down that you're not honoring your commitment to conscious, deliberate decision making. This shakes your food freedom foundation and makes it far more likely that you'll say, "What the hell" and order dessert, too, whether you want it or not.

Let's fix this scenario.

Happy birthday! You have plans with friends at your favorite restaurant tonight, and you're excited to celebrate with them. You have no preconceived expectations about what you'll order, because you're committed to making conscious, deliberate, "worth it" decisions in the moment, birthday or not. You recognize the evening isn't about the food or drink—it's about sharing this special day with people you care about.

You arrive at the restaurant and open the drink menu. Is anything here worth it in this minute? Will wine or a martini mess you up? Do you really want it? You decide then and there, based on how you feel in the moment, and order in a way that honors your intentions.

You happily toast to your birthday with your friends (does it really matter what's in your glass?), feeling totally satisfied with your choice. You repeat this process as you consider your appetizer, main course, and dessert.

By the end of the meal, you've ordered only the things you truly wanted, you've savored every bite, you've celebrated with people you care about, and you leave the restaurant feeling confident and in control. Plus, you may have twelve extra dollars in your pocket.

That's a pretty good birthday, if you ask me.

In summary, as part of your Food Freedom plan, *you can have anything you want, any time you darn well please.* Reminding yourself of this takes an enormous amount of pressure off you in that immediate situation. If you truly embrace this concept in the moment, it will be easier to walk away from something you don't really want, and far less likely that you'll mindlessly hoover something that's not worth it, just because it's a holiday or special occasion.

Trigger #4: Stress

In the last chapter, you learned that stress can drain even the most substantial willpower bank and, left unchecked for too long, will always promote cravings. This, unfortunately, is the opposite of good news for your food freedom. Many highly stressful events—think divorces, funerals, the postpartum Twilight Zone—are littered with junk and comfort food.

During times of immense stress, it's good to accept this. Placing unrealistic expectations on yourself ("I won't give in to cravings"; "I'll make my diet perfect"; "I'll never stress eat") only creates more stress, rendering your cravings even harder to resist. Do yourself a favor by acknowledging that certain healthy practices are likely to slip during difficult times. This will alleviate some pressure and help you create a more realistic picture of what life will look like in the coming days, weeks, or months.

On the other hand, that's no excuse to completely throw in the towel, invoking the ultimate WTH Effect: "I'm so stressed, I'm just going to do whatever I want right now to make myself feel better." How well has that strategy worked in the past to keep you healthy, happy, and gracefully coping? Wait, I'll tell you.

It has not worked well.

If your stress is really short term (like a big exam tomorrow), it's probably not a big deal if you indulge in pizza and soda tonight while you stay up late studying. But in the case of ongoing stress, the minute you give in to this idea, you've already lost. When stressors are ongoing, doing whatever you want also creates more stress, as you overconsume, gain weight, lose self-confidence, and feel so out of control and guilty that you just eat more.

In summary, neither of these approaches—aiming for perfection or throwing in the towel—are particularly effective. So let's try something else:

creating a plan for dealing with stressful situations, using some of the tools you've already learned.

KNOWN STRESSORS: If the stress is known (a new baby on the way, a planned cross-country move, a job change), start thinking well ahead of time about how you can stockpile some healthy behaviors to give yourself a cushion once the stress hits. It doesn't work quite this neatly in the body, of course—stress is still stress, and there is no "get out of jail free" card that you can earn now and play later. But going into it with a buffer of healthy behaviors, self-control, and self-confidence will accomplish the big-picture goal: preventing total burnout and allowing you to bounce back in a few weeks, instead of a few months.

EXTRA CREDIT

Preparing for tough times is like taking on every extra credit assignment in school. You build up points now so if you can't study as much later in the semester or don't perform as well on exams, you've got an insurance policy. Your grades may slip, but thanks to the extra credit points, they'll only drop to a C instead of an F.

This always starts with your diet, for two reasons. First, your nutrition has a profound impact on your health and how well you're able to manage stress. If you're underfed and undernourished, you're far less resilient, and the goal here is to make you strong and all-around healthy heading into the stressful situation.

Second, one stressful event can make you feel like *everything* in your life is spinning out of control. You can't dictate your new baby's temperament, how much sleep you'll be able to cobble together, your toddler's reaction to the new addition, or whether visitors will drop in unexpectedly. . . but you can always control the food you put in your mouth. Every day, you have the opportunity to exert some influence over your environment and gain confidence in your ability to handle your business by making dietary choices that make you healthier.

I'm not suggesting you set unreasonable expectations. I'm not insisting you win every battle with your Sugar Dragon. Just commit to feeding yourself well during this difficult time, so you're better prepared to handle what needs handling, and can emerge from the stress bent but not broken.

Ideally, this means doing another reset leading up to the event.* Just as you do pre-holiday or pre-vacation, you want to boost your health and remind yourself that you feel and perform your best when you're eating a healthy diet. This will strengthen your self-confidence, and help you at least delay the arrival of your Sugar Dragon once the stress starts rolling in. Time your reset to end at least ten days before the anticipated big day, so you aren't trying to manage reintroduction during a business trip with your new boss or midnight feedings with the baby.

Then, in the thick of the storm, just do your best. The most important thing to remember during stressful times, especially when it comes to your diet:

Let good enough be good enough.

Buy pre-made grilled salmon and kale salad from the health food store yet again. Reheat chicken sausage and leftover veggies for the fourth time this week. Skip recipes and pile healthy ingredients you happen to have on hand on a plate . . . and make it a paper plate, because doing dishes is not at the top of your list right now.

This is good enough.

Are you eating the most nutritious, well-rounded, Pinterest-worthy meals you could have made? No. Do they exactly follow your ideal meal template? No. Could you have put more effort into your meals? Sure.

But . . .

Are you sticking to a healthy diet? YES. Are you leaning on junk food or comfort food because you're stressed and unprepared? NO. Are these meals good enough for what is happening in your life right now? SO MUCH YES.

In this context, where so many of your resources are devoted to simply surviving this difficult time gracefully, *let this be enough*. Make yourself resilient by eating the foods you've decided are healthiest for you. Show yourself grace if and when you give in to cravings. Remember: You've got a solid plan for getting back on track once this stressful time is over, so don't worry about that now. Take some of the pressure off here, because you're already dealing with more than enough.

This, too, shall pass. Amen.

When your stressful time is over, take stock and ask yourself, "Where am I now?" If your energy is in the tank, your Sugar Dragon is roaring, your

* If you're pregnant and considering a reset, visit the Healthy Mama, Happy Baby website (mamas.whole30.com) for our specific pregnancy recommendations.

self-confidence could use a boost, or your symptoms are flaring, return immediately to your reset (see chapter 10). If you didn't go too far off the rails, simply continue with your Food Freedom plan, putting extra effort into preparing more creative meals and using a wider variety of foods to restore excitement to your taste buds. Or do something in between: If you don't want a full reset but feel like a mini reset or a few additional rules (like "No dessert for a month") would help, just do that. You get to decide what you need post-stress to return to a place where you feel strong and in control, but this time, you're not going it alone—you've got your Food Freedom plan and experience backing you up.

SHRINK YOUR WORLD

One big-picture strategy I employ during stressful times is shrinking my world down so it's more manageable. During time-sensitive work projects, for example, I'll spend a month doing nothing but writing, sleeping, and exercising. That means I accept no family visitors, make really simple (but still healthy) meals, don't socialize often, and generally lead a boring life, but that's exactly what helps me get through the tough time. If I were to try to fit it all in while devoting extra attention to my work, I'd quickly exhaust my willpower and energy reserves. So I narrow my focus, retain what's most important to me during this time, and end up coming out of the craziness just as healthy as I was going into it. During your stressful time, prioritize the three things that are the most important given your context (work, exercise, sleep, friends, family), and accept that the rest will be sacrificed for the greater good until you can catch your breath.

SUDDEN STRESS: Unfortunately, stress sometimes blindsides you, like when there's a death in the family or you're abruptly laid off from your job. When stress comes upon you suddenly, you're at an obvious disadvantage. (All the more reason to manage stress from a big-picture perspective, so you're never depleted to the point where a life crisis will totally destroy your health.) You obviously cannot plan a reset before this type of event, as you didn't know it was coming, so you'll have to decide how to handle your dietary plan on the fly.

That may or may not include a return to your reset diet.

To reset or not to reset during an unforeseen stressful period is something only you can decide. For some, returning to the rules of the reset will feel soothing and stress relieving, taking some big decisions out of your hands and allowing you to conserve willpower during this already hectic time. This generally applies to people for whom the reset rules feel easy and effortless, and who have been staying within their definition of "food freedom" for long enough that the reset won't feel that different. However, if you're new to this program, haven't reset in a while, or haven't been working your Food Freedom plan, the pressure of following the rules could be the stress-straw that breaks your craving-camel's back.

Use this trick to figure out the right strategy for you:

FIRST, PICTURE YOUR LIFE ON THE RESET. Do you imagine yourself feeling happier, more in control, and able to take the energy you would be spending on dietary decisions and apply it elsewhere? Do you see how the self-confidence a reset brings will spill over into other areas of your life, helping you more effectively manage stress? Or do you feel even more stressed, overwhelmed by the rules, exhausted by the preparations, and frustrated because your favorite healthy convenience foods are out because of a gram of added sugar?

NOW PICTURE THE SAME STRESSFUL CIRCUMSTANCES OFF THE RESET. Do you see yourself eating popcorn and wine for dinner, comforting yourself with candy and cookies, feeling tired and cranky; more depressed, anxious, and stressed than ever? Or do you feel relieved because there's one less thing to worry about, still confident that you can balance a healthy-enough eating plan with everything else going on in your life?

If doing a reset during this difficult time will provide you with the healthy foundation you need to handle your stress more effectively, then get back on it as soon as you're prepared to. Stick to it until things calm down, and let the sense of self-control, improved energy, better sleep, and brighter outlook it brings see you through this difficult time.

If, however, life on the reset seems daunting and needlessly demanding, then skip it for now. The pressures of a formal reset are going to do more harm than good in your context, so don't do that to yourself. Simply commit to a healthy, balanced plan with as much intent of awareness and conscientious decision-making as you can muster, and follow the "let good enough be good enough" advice on page 144.

Whether your stress was expected or a shock, once it has eased enough for you to feel ready, it's time for another reset. First, you'll need the major health benefits a reset brings, because even if your diet didn't totally jump the shark, your health has certainly been compromised. (In some cases, the ongoing stress response can be more damaging than the stressor itself.) Second, a reset brings a sense of self-control that will spill over into other areas of your life, helping you restore order where stress may have knocked things off-kilter. Finally, more restful sleep and increased energy will encourage you to return to other healthy practices, like exercise, meditation, or socialization, that may have temporarily gone on walkabout.

BEWARE OF BOOZE

While you're probably more tempted than ever to turn to wine or other alcohol for comfort during this stressful time, do your best to resist. Alcohol numbs you in the moment, yes, but it will only exacerbate your stress by disrupting your sleep, depleting micronutrients, impairing your gut, and firing up your immune system. Alcohol can also contribute to feelings of depression and anxiety—something you really don't need right now. Even if you're not up for a full or partial reset during this difficult time, it would be very wise to institute a "no booze" rule. Bonus: This will also help you stay true to your healthy-eating intentions, as you're more likely to make poor, impulsive food choices if you're a few glasses deep.

Trigger #5: Home Alone

Many people find that their food choices swiftly take a turn into kid-in-a-candy-store when there's no on there to witness it or hold them accountable. For some, this leads to out-of-control eating or binging; for others, it just brings a slightly unbridled feeling and more off-plan choices than usual. Why is it so common to face-plant into a bag of potato chips when you're home alone?

First, there's something about being home alone that makes you feel like a pre-teen left without a babysitter for the very first time. It's so exciting!

No one is watching! You can do anything you want! You can have pizza and beer for dinner and stay up late eating ice cream while binge-watching *Million Dollar Listing* and NO ONE WILL JUDGE YOU.

I swear, this is universal. It doesn't matter whether you're 22 or 52; when you're used to living with other people and then find yourself home alone, you turn into your 12-year-old self. But with money. And a car. And more expensive taste in comfort food. (Think a 2009 Beaujolais and Madagascar dark chocolate instead of a slushee and Cool Ranch Doritos.)

In addition, being home alone can be stressful if the unaccompanied time is unwanted or unexpected. Maybe you're single-parenting while your spouse is gone, or used to your partner doing the bulk of the grocery shopping and cooking. You may feel lonely, missing the companionship. Many women say that being home alone is a little scary and causes them poor sleep and anxiety. As you now know, it's normal to see an increase in cravings when you're under stress, especially if the current stress of being home alone is on top of chronic stress. It's no wonder your trips to the pantry increase if your solo status is more anxiety inducing than liberating.

Finally, there's one more reason we tend to slow-slide back into less healthy habits when we find ourselves home alone:

Plain old laziness.

Without anyone else to cook for (or eat with), you may just decide to take it easy and skip the shopping, meal prep, and cooking. Which is totally fine—a rotisserie chicken plus a trip to the salad bar is quick, easy, and gets the job done. But often, a slide from recipes to ingredient meals slips further into "I'll just get Chinese/eat dark chocolate and a block of cheddar/go out" when you're home alone. And that laziness, especially combined with not having a dining companion, spells trouble for your new healthy habits.

Here, again, your best defense is a good offense. Before your housemate's next trip, make a list of all the ways you can relish your alone time without gorging on less-healthy food. Walk around in your underwear. Take a long, uninterrupted bath. Cook a fancy dinner and eat in peace and quiet in a leisurely fashion. Watch a movie while sprawled on the couch, slip in bed at 7:30 p.m. to read a good book, or reorganize a living space on your own terms.

Once your housemate leaves, take a moment to luxuriate in your aloneness, but also practice something I call the "I'm an adult" affirmation. Remind yourself that you are a grown-up person who can legitimately eat whatever you want, whenever you want. Take some of the "specialness" out of this situation, at least when it comes to your food, and you may find the teenage rebel in you is placated by the idea that there's nothing *actually* rebellious about eating ice cream at this stage in your life.

From a practical perspective, get rid of the stuff in your house that may tempt you to binge. If your housemates will want it when they return, make it way less accessible; stuff it in a bottom drawer, move it to the back of the freezer, or ask them to hide it in an out-of-the-way location. Then, first thing in the morning when willpower is strongest, draft a meal plan for the week and grocery shop for just those items. Do that, and you'll be adhering to an incredibly important food freedom tip—one that applies to far more scenarios than this "home alone" tale:

If you don't have it, you can't eat it.

Resisting cravings for things you don't really want or aren't really worth it starts in the grocery store. The sheer anticipation of something sweet, salty, fatty, or crunchy going in your cart is enough to stimulate dopamine, the "wanting" neurotransmitter. If you're shopping while distracted, hungry, stressed, or emotional, it's all too easy to toss these less-healthy comfort foods in your cart. You'll think, "It's not like I'll *definitely* eat this tube of cookie dough. I'm buying it . . . just in case." But we both know that's a lie. Cravings Airlines Flight 103 is landing right on schedule, and it's taxiing directly toward your pie-hole.

Buying a rewarding, tempting treat is as good as eating it, so if you can commit to shopping carefully and deliberately from your list, applying as much awareness to the things you *buy* as the things you *eat*, you'll save yourself a ton of willpower energy when you get home. Let's illustrate with a story. P. G. of Utah instituted a rule around ice cream after his first Whole30: As part of his Food Freedom plan, he doesn't buy ice cream for home, but will enjoy some if he's out and it's being served. This greatly reduces his ice cream temptation, helps him conserve willpower, and makes this special treat even more special.

Let's say P. G. has been successful at the grocery store and leaves without a pint of Chunky Monkey in his cart. That means, should a craving hit at 10 p.m., he'll have to go through a major to-do in order to satisfy it: talk himself into leaving the house late at night, change out of his pajamas, find his shoes, find his keys, and warm up the car to drive to the 7-Eleven. But remember, the average craving lasts just *three to five minutes*. Somewhere in the middle of all his preparations, P. G. will notice that his craving has subsided and he can escape unscathed (except perhaps feeling silly that he actually considered leaving the house in the middle of the night for something called Chunky Monkey).

IF YOU BINGE

I've worked with clients with a serious history of binging when left home alone. This behavior is incredibly damaging both physically and psychologically. If this is your context, you can buy yourself an extra insurance policy with "if/then" plans for potentially difficult moments. These plans might sound a little too extreme for the average home-aloner, but if you're desperate to break this cycle, take this step seriously. Create a plan with your counselor or therapist, write it down, and post it in a conspicuous place while you're home alone. Refer back to it as often as needed, adding additional "if/then" scenarios as you think of them.

IF . . .	THEN . . .
you find yourself having serious cravings,	you'll phone a friend/do the dishes/curl up with a good book/take a bath.
you're at the grocery store feeling tempted,	you'll pull out your list and follow your own instructions/leave the store and come back later/ jump on social media and put out a call for help.
you find yourself eating less-healthy food in an out-of-control fashion while home alone,	you'll contact your counselor/go to the gym or outside for a walk/call your partner or spouse for some reassurance.

Getting through this situation unscathed just once with assistance from your new food freedom tools will help you build the confidence you need to break this pattern once and for all, and reinforce your growth mind-set: "I am a healthy person, even when no one is watching."

It's Okay to Slip

Last but not least, remember that your food freedom path isn't going to be one long line of linear progress. Don't beat yourself up if your habits slip when your situation changes, especially if you're a creature of routine. Awareness is the first step in keeping yourself on an even keel when you find yourself sliding back into less-healthy habits. Making a plan is the next. The more you practice creating new routines, reducing stress, exercising your "worth it" skills, and managing cravings during these challenging times, the smoother your food freedom sailing will feel in everyday life.

Also, you should talk about this part. This isn't Fight Club: The first rule of slipping is *not* "Don't talk about slipping."

Share the challenges you're facing with family, friends, or a trusted counselor, because talking about it serves more than one purpose. Bringing something you used to feel ashamed of (eating less-healthy food) out into the open reminds you that there is nothing here to feel bad about—you're just struggling and need some help. Saying it out loud can also help you see your situation more clearly; perhaps you'll come up with the right fix on the spot. "Now that I'm talking about it, I see that this only really happens when my roommate goes to bed early and I'm downstairs by myself. I bet it would help if I created a nighttime ritual that doesn't involve food." Finally, sharing your food freedom journey—the ups and the downs—with others brings you closer together, and enables them to better support your efforts.

Still, if all your in-the-moment and big-picture strategies can't get you back to where you'd like to be, you're okay. You have a plan. And if you follow it, I promise it will work.

If all else fails, you can always fall back to your reset.

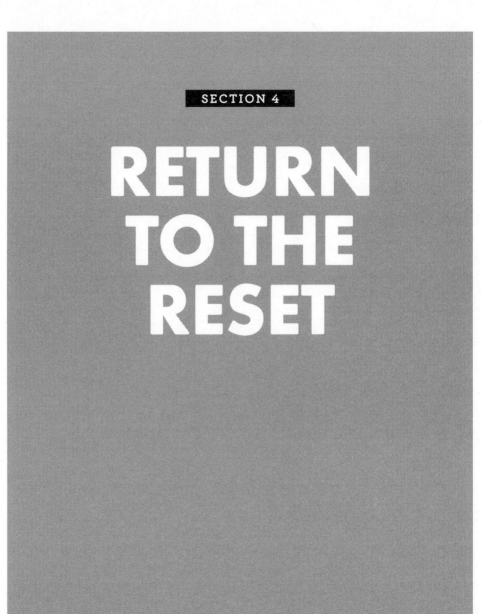

SECTION 4

RETURN TO THE RESET

CHAPTER 10

BACK TO THE START

Blogger and certified group fitness trainer Shannon C. was a Whole30 success story, sharing her non-scale victories and reset advice with her clients and audience. For six months, she rather effortlessly enjoyed her food freedom. But the latter part of 2014 brought a busload of stress: client demands, relationship issues, a hospitalized family member, and an automobile accident that left her with bruises, a swollen knee, and mounds of paperwork and insurance red tape. Shannon found herself veering off her food freedom path with sweets and dairy, letting comfort foods slip back into her diet on a regular basis. She tried to rein it in on her own, but her failure to successfully moderate only led to even more unhealthy choices. After a few months of stress-eating, she was struggling with energy, sleeping poorly, and feeling bloated and out of control.

While Shannon leaned heavily on her faith during these tough times, she knew another reset was the best way to put herself back in the driver's seat. "With so much uncertainty and stress in my life, the Whole30 reset gave me *something* I could control and succeed with," Shannon explains. Once she returned to her reset, she found a sense of comfort and order in the familiarity of the rules and structure, and other healthy habits fell back into place. As she puts it, "When so many other unfamiliar stresses were weighing on me, returning to my reset actually lifted the burden and put me back in control."

While the techniques outlined in Chapter 9 are designed to help you spot your triggers and keep you from straying too far off the food freedom path, it's good to have a backup strategy in case you find yourself lost in the forest with a fire-breathing Sugar Dragon on your tail. Even the best-laid plans can go awry, and any one of those last four triggers (especially when combined with a gradual slow slide back into old habits) may prove difficult to recover from gracefully. The good news is that you already have a proven plan to regain food freedom, no matter how out-of-control you may once again find yourself feeling. Just go back to your reset.

There. Don't you feel better already?

THE 80/20 RULE

Robert Sapolsky, professor of biology and neurology at Stanford University, proposes that 80 percent of stress reduction can be attributed to the first 20 percent of effort. It's why you feel so relieved just by making an appointment with a counselor, signing up to join a gym, or ordering that book on meditation. You haven't actually *done* anything yet, but your brain likes that you've taken the first step and translates that into stress relief. Sometimes, this can backfire—you'll feel so much better that you'll want to check this task off your list altogether. To combat that, you're going to commit to your reset—then follow it through using the techniques outlined in this chapter.

If you feel in need of an intervention at any point in your food freedom journey, simply return to your preferred reset. (Or, if part of the reason you're here is because the design-your-own option didn't work very well for you, commit to something a little more robust, like the Whole30.) Start the process all the way over from the beginning by committing to the reset; going public to gain accountability and support; getting prepared with a pantry clean-out, meal plan, and grocery shopping; preparing for potentially challenging situations; and . . . GO.

RETURNING TO THE RESET

- Come back to the reset as often as necessary.

- Do this for as long as necessary to feel 100% back in control.

- Reintroduce.

- Return to enjoying your food freedom.

It's as simple as that.

You know it works. You know it will feel great. You know it will restore your self-confidence, self-control, and happiness. So do it, and get back to that place where your energy is rocking, skin is glowing, cravings are banished, and a healthy, sustainable balance is back within your grasp. Complete another reset, learn even more about how food affects you with another careful reintroduction, and take all that information with you to build an even more robust foundation for your ongoing food freedom. This reset will automatically delay the advent of another slow slide; give you clarity to make an even better holiday, vacation, or home-alone plan; and provide you with even more tools and practice to gracefully manage stress.

It's so easy it almost feels like cheating.

When It's Not Easy

Except sometimes, you feel stuck. Sometimes, you know you should do something, and you know you'd feel so much better if you *just did it* . . . and yet you can't. Something keeps you from taking that first step, even though logically, you really want to and you know it will help. It's like you've got a really big interview to get to, but your car is stuck in Park, and you can't figure out how to get it into Drive, no matter how desperately you want to start moving.

Feeling stuck is the worst.

You know you need to get back to your reset. Every day you tell yourself, "Today is the day," and every day you find a new excuse to put it off. You're mad at yourself for not doing what you know you need to do. You're mad at the people you see actually doing it while you aren't. You're mad at me for saying, "JUST DO THE THING ALREADY," when you've TRIED and you CAN'T. You're just *mad*, and that state of mind is only feeding your Sugar Dragon, who thrives on a diet of anger and frustration.

Something is preventing you from starting your reset engine.

I'm not a psychologist, so I won't get into the idea that people do things for a reason, and if there wasn't an emotional payoff, you wouldn't keep doing it. (Although I think there's something to be said for working through this stuff with a trained counselor, especially if getting "stuck" is a pattern that pops up frequently in your life.) I will, however, help you feel less crazy for not being able to just do the thing already.

You're not actually crazy. It's the food.

You've been inhaling calorically dense, nutritionally sparse, super-rewarding comfort foods like it's your full-time job since that holiday/vacation/stressful event (or for no good reason—you just have been). Overconsuming these "foods with no brakes"—the stuff that once you start eating, you can't stop eating—causes a cascade of physical and mental consequences, all of which make it really hard for you to break the cycle and get back to your reset.

- These scientist-designed, carbohydrate-rich, calorie-dense foods combine sugar, salt, and fat in amounts not seen in nature, stimulating your brain with giant hits of pleasure and reward.

- Your brain worships at the altar of pleasure and reward, so it reinforces habit loops designed to promote cravings for even more sugar, salt, and fat.

- These cravings are really hard to ignore (thanks, dopamine), so you give in even when you're not hungry, and especially when you're anxious, lonely, bored, or tired.

- Since most of the micronutrients, fiber, water, protein, and fat have been processed out of these foods, your body gets lots of calories but still doesn't feel nourished—so you overconsume.

- This puts you on a blood sugar roller coaster; the ensuing energy spikes and crashes driving more sugar cravings and moving you back toward a metabolic reliance on sugar instead of fat.

- Emotionally, you're back in the same craving → overconsumption → guilt → shame → remorse cycle that feels all too familiar, the stress of which (guess what?) promotes cravings.

And all the while, you're sitting in your driveway with the keys in the engine, crying into a box of cinnamon buns and listening to "Everybody Hurts" on repeat.

I'm not saying you're not responsible, because unless someone ties you up and force-feeds you Oreos, you've made the choices that led you to this place. But understand one thing: *These foods are designed to make you crave them and built specifically for overconsumption.* You're not crazy—you're just responding exactly the way food scientists knew you would.

Do you feel a little better now? Good.

Now take a deep breath and put on your big-girl (or -boy) pants, because you're about to get to work. You're not actually stuck; you're just freaked out. The idea of going from where you are now to Day 31 of a successful reset is exhausting. Looking even farther down your food freedom road is even more overwhelming. You begin thinking about how well you were doing and how far you've slipped, imagining the long trek ahead of you. It's like you're staring up at the biggest hill you've ever seen, and you're wearing roller skates. With wheels made of donuts. Tasty, tasty donuts.

Your inner monologue probably sounds like this: "I was doing so well, but now I'm back where I started. It's going to be such hard work to feel awesome again. Can I even feel that awesome again? Will it always be this hard? Will I ever find my balance? I hate where I am, but I just can't move forward."*

Let's move you forward.

You're going to steal a mantra taken straight out of 12-step recovery programs. Groups like Alcoholics Anonymous or Overeaters Anonymous have plenty of proven success strategies under their belts, including the popular phrase "One day at a time." And that's how you're going to get back to your reset, feeling awesome, and food freedom: one day, one meal, one bite at a time. So right now, ask yourself just one question:

"What's the very next thing I have to do to get back to my reset?"

I'll help you by breaking down the "one day at a time" motto even further. Shifting your food freedom car out of Park starts with just *one meal*, and using whatever tricks you can to stay present and not project too far ahead of yourself.

---

* Sounds like your growth mind-set has also taken a backseat to old habits and negative self-talk. Don't worry about this now—that will be easy to restore once you've recommitted to your reset.

Today Is Your Day 1

Yes, now. Right now. With your next bite of food, you're back on your reset. I know you have food in your house that is compliant. Start eating it. But here's the psychological trick . . .

It's just one meal. You only have to go back to your reset for ONE MEAL. You can wrap your head around that—one reset-worthy meal. The meal *after* that can be vodka and ice cream sandwiches if you want . . . but *this* meal is 100% compliant.

Proceed. Cook yourself some good food. Enjoy it. Allow yourself to feel the satisfaction that comes from doing something so incredibly healthy. High-five yourself for a job well done. Then repeat this same strategy for each and every meal. Tell yourself that just for this meal, you're going to make it reset-friendly. The next meal doesn't have to be, but *this* meal is a reset meal.

The logical side of you is saying, "But wait, what if for the next meal, I really DO want vodka and ice cream sandwiches?" That's the trick. Because even if you do, you're still going to tell yourself to get through one more meal before throwing in the towel. Again and again, it's just one more meal . . . and even though you intuitively know you're tricking yourself, *it will work*.

Because science.

The fact that you're giving yourself permission to go off the plan with the next meal removes a huge amount of pressure. You won't feel trapped in a 30-day reset, contemplating how you'll get through 90 reset meals in a row; you're just focusing on one. It takes advantage of the "status quo" bias: your emotional preference to keep doing what you're already doing. It breaks your goal down into something manageable, but it also accomplishes a critical task: it gives you a huge sense of accomplishment. If 80 percent of your stress can be mitigated with the first 20 percent of effort, you've just taken a huge step toward breaking your return-to-reset paralysis. And that's gonna feel so good, you'll be able to continue in this fashion for the next meal. And the next. And the next.

Although at some point, you're going to need to grocery shop.

Repeat this process one meal at a time, and you'll quickly realize that you're actually cruising up the reset freeway. By now, you've distanced yourself from the empty reward of fatty, sugary, salty comfort foods; begun to correct blood sugar regulation and restore hormonal balance; and given yourself a break from the emotional roller coaster you've been riding. Once you've sufficiently distanced yourself from the cravings, you can stop doing your little trick at every meal. (Or keep doing it for every meal, if it helps. Personally, this is one of my favorite motivational tools when I'm trying to change a habit.)

ONE DAY, ONE MEAL, ONE BITE AT A TIME

Whole30er Michelle K. of Katy, Texas, uses this tactic get through stress-related p.m. cravings. She says, "Night is the worst time for me, so I tell myself that if I can finish this day sticking to my healthy plan, then tomorrow I can do whatever I want. The next morning, I am so happy I am another day further into my food freedom journey that I find I just want to keep going. I realized if I can honor the commitment I made to myself and push through the day or moment, then I can come back at a better time and truly decide if this action is something I want to pursue."

Most of you will need a full reset to get back on track, especially if you're new to the Food Freedom plan, or if it's been a very long time since your last reset (and you've been a very naughty monkey between now and then). That means a minimum of 30 days, plus the full reintroduction period. When you're feeling seriously out of control, Sugar Dragon roaring, energy and blood sugar fluctuating like a roller coaster . . . now is not the time for shortcuts.

There *still* aren't any quick fixes. It will be hard work (again). But the more you practice, the easier it gets; it's totally worth it, as you'll remember from your first reset; and getting back there is not as hard as you've made it out to be in your head. You know what works, and you know how to do it. So just do it—but don't allow yourself to be overwhelmed. Get back on the road one mile (wait, meal) at a time, until your cravings and negative self-talk are just a speck in your rearview mirror.

The Role of a Mini Reset

For some people and in the right circumstances, an abbreviated reset can be an appropriate tool to keep you on the food freedom path. If you've got lots of experience with your reset and stay pretty close to your ideal diet otherwise, it may only take you a week to jump straight to "tiger blood," where you're feeling energetic, confident, and back in control. In that case, there's no need to always extend your reset to the full 30 days just to say you did. Food freedom demands that you live by your own rules as often as possible, so don't follow a strict reset any longer than you really need to.

There are a number of circumstances in which a mini reset may be the right tool for the job. Maybe your Sugar Dragon has just barely started to awaken, and you feel like a quick Craving Reset will send it back to sleep. Or you have a big presentation or exam coming up, and you want to look and feel your best heading into it. Some people just throw in a mini reset regularly for good measure, 5 to 10 days at a time, as a preemptive way to keep their healthy food freedom habits solidly in place.

If you get to Day 7 or Day 10 and realize you're not where you want to be, just keep going. Turning your mini reset into a full reset because you're further away from food freedom than you thought isn't a strategic failure—it's just another learning experience. Figuring out how many days you need to be feeling amazing again is a good way to track progress; if you need 25 days this go-round, but the next mini reset has you growling like a tiger by Day 14, that's great news.

ALL OF THE BAD, NONE OF THE GOOD

All you naughty monkeys from the last section are now thinking, "Wait, a mini reset? I'll take that, please!" Hear me clearly: If you've gone pretty far off the rails since your last reset, are still new to food freedom, or your medical condition or symptoms are presenting again, an abbreviated reset will do you more harm than good. Think back to your first reset. How much fun were the first ten days? Yeah, not that fun. Resetting for 5, 7, or even 14 days is probably just long enough to remind you how hard the first half of a reset can be but not long enough to have you seeing the magic—a serious lose-lose situation. If this is your context, do yourself and your body a favor and reboot for the whole 30 days.

Still reintroduce. Always reintroduce. Remember, reintroduction is a lifelong experience, and even a mini reset is a great opportunity to see how things work in the context of your newly reestablished "clean slate."

Finally, the guidelines for a mini reset are the exactly same as those of a full-length program. Resist temptation to relax on the rules, cut corners, or allow common triggers like sugar or alcohol into the reset because you "know" they work for you. Every reset is another opportunity to learn even more about how potentially problematic foods impact your body, habits, and emotional relationship with food. The only thing different here is the time frame.

Wash, Rinse, Repeat

Returning to your reset is an important part of your Food Freedom plan; a foolproof "get back in control" strategy meant to be employed as often as you feel is necessary. It will likely feel necessary more frequently in the beginning. This is okay. You're working hard to reprogram habits, break unhealthy associations, and learn a whole new language around food. Much like anyone trying to quit smoking or improve their health, there is no shame in needing support and help along the way.

Part of my recovery included regular group counseling sessions and meetings. In the beginning, I attended several a week; I needed all the support I could get while trying to change my addictive behaviors. As I grew more comfortable in my new healthy habits, better able to manage cravings and stress using the tools I had learned, I relied less and less on meetings, and only attended when things were especially hard or I was struggling more than usual.

These meetings were my "reset," a safe space where I could recommit, gain support, and leave feeling confident and back in control. I never felt bad about needing them. On the contrary, I was proud of myself for accepting the extra help, and comforted that I had something I knew I could return to whenever I needed it to keep me on track.

Returning to your reset is neither a failure nor a weakness.

Changing something as emotional as your relationship with food is hard. You've gathered many tools to help you stay committed, focused, and in control as you navigate this food freedom journey. Think of your reset as just another tool. If you need the extra support, it will always be there for you. Use it when you need it, gaining confidence from each and every revisit. And remember that admitting you need help during a difficult time is a sign of strength, and a *huge* indicator of the progress you've made.

After all, your cries for help used to look a lot like sticking your face into a pint of frozen yogurt.

TOUGH LOVE

t's time for some more tough love. Think of your reset as a safety net, there for you as you venture out on your own food freedom balance beam. You'll walk, balance, feel great . . . and slip. Which may shake you up a little, but does no real harm, because the safety net is there to catch you. However, a safety net does not equal permission to ride a unicycle while juggling flaming cupcakes on your balance beam. Translation: Just because you know the reset is there to help you get back on track does not excuse you from staying conscious and aware, and making deliberate decisions while you're practicing food freedom. It's a just-in-case safety net, not a trampoline. Besides, bouncing back to your reset too often isn't fun, isn't healthy, and isn't actually freedom.

How often you should reset is highly variable, based on your needs, how far you are into the process, and how much you love the comfort and surety of following your reset rules. Some choose to reset themselves on a regular schedule, just as they check their carbon monoxide detectors or turn the clocks forward or back every spring and fall. Others will return to their reset simply to support their spouse or a co-worker taking it on for the first time. I prefer to schedule them only as needed. I've done a full Whole30 twice in one year, but for the last two years, I've been able to keep my food freedom on track with only the occasional Whole7 or Whole14.

There are pros and cons to all these approaches, so let's walk through them to help you make a better decision about when, why, and how to incorporate various reset possibilities into your life. I'll summarize my best recommendations for you to follow, until you're comfortable enough to create your own reset timeline.

REGULARLY SCHEDULED RESETS

PROS:

- Keeps you on track, even if you've slipped and are hesitant to admit it.

- Keeps you better connected with your healthy-eating community, which provides you with ongoing motivation and support.

- Ensures you'll regularly continue to increase awareness around how less-healthy foods impact you.

CONS:

- May be hard to fully commit if you don't feel like you need it.

- May tempt you to go off the rails pre-reset, since you know a cleanup is coming.

- Too frequent resets feel less like food freedom, because you're not spending enough time finding your own balance

RESETTING WITH FAMILY OR FRIENDS

PROS:

- Unexpected resets on someone else's timeline really help keep you on track.

- Brings you closer with family and friends; gives you more in-person support.

- Sharing your healthy eating journey with others will deepen your commitment to your own.

CONS:

- May be hard to fully commit if you don't feel like you need it.

- If your family/friend struggles, complains, or quits, it may weaken your own resolve in the moment.

RESETTING WHEN YOU DECIDE YOU NEED IT

PROS:

- Ensures you are fully committed to each and every reset.

- Forces you to stay present and aware with your habits and acknowledge when you've slipped; a good practice.

- Allows you to enjoy your food freedom for as long as you can successfully manage it—which could be a long time.

CONS:

- May find yourself off the rails for a longer period of time, reluctant to admit you've slipped.

- Will be emotionally and physically harder to come back to if you wait too long.

My Reset Recommendations

To give you a little more guidance, here are my best big-picture recommendations based on the pros and cons of the approaches I outlined in chapter 4, and what I've observed within the Whole30 community. This is a great place to start if you're new to the Food Freedom plan, but many Whole30ers have successfully followed this same strategy for years.

- Schedule one annual reset each year; I highly recommend a start date of January 1. Nearly everyone needs a little help recovering from the holiday season, and because so many people will choose to reset at this time, support and resources will be widely available.

- If a friend, family member, or co-worker wants to try a reset, consider whether you need to do it with them to be supportive. If you're secure in and enjoying your food freedom, remember you can help them just as much by being their daily check-in or helping them plan their meals.

- Practice your food freedom skills, and at the earliest sign of needing help (feeling out of control, and not being able to regain control using the other tools provided), recommit to a reset.

NOW A WORD ON YO-YO RESETS. If, before reading this book, you vacillated between strict dieting and falling off the wagon hard, I hope the advice you've picked up here has helped pull you out of that cycle. But if after a few food freedom cycles, you still find yourself ping-ponging between "I'm on a reset!" and "I'm knee-deep in a box of Cronuts," there's obviously something that needs addressing. Ask yourself a few questions:

- Are you still thinking about this like a DIET, where you restrict, starve, and white-knuckle your way through until it "ends"? *Solution:* Reread page 60 and remind yourself *this* is not *that*.

- Are you getting lazy in your worth-it evaluations or skipping over the short-term and long-term food freedom success strategies? *Solution:* Recommit to the material in chapters 7 and 8, because until you start practicing, these will never become a habit.

- Are you thinking of your reset as penance for your less-healthy eating? Yes, it's a safety net, but using it to "make up for" poor, impulsive, or lazy decisions around food is old dieting mentality.

Solution: Reread the tough love on page 164, and remember you can't "crash reset" like you used to "crash diet."

- Are you being too hard on yourself, or expecting too much too soon? *Solution:* Show yourself some grace. Know that over time and with dedication to the process, these habits *will* stick, and you'll be on the Food Freedom path for longer and longer stretches of time—but it doesn't happen overnight, and slips *are* expected.

- Do you have deeper unresolved emotional issues around food? *Solution:* The Food Freedom plan alone can't bring everyone to a healthy relationship with food. Recruit the help of a reputable counselor or psychologist to explore what is keeping you stuck in this cycle.

Second Time's a Charm?

Now that you're comfortable with the idea of returning to your reset whenever you need it, there's something else I need to warn you about.

The second reset may be harder than the first.

In fact, for those who come back for a second round of the Whole30, more than 1 in 4 will find the second one even more challenging.*

Not what you were expecting, I know.

You're all, "How can this be? I'm a label-reading maniac, I know the rules of the reset inside and out, and I have a support network of Instagram friends and forum buddies to help keep me on track. I make my own mayo and don't even own a scale anymore, for goodness' sake. So why would the second round be *harder?*"

Because reasons, that's why. A few of them. But the good news is that all of them are foreseeable, preventable, or at the very least manageable. Let's dig in.

THE NEWNESS IS GONE. The first reason is simple: Your reset is no longer a bright, shiny toy. While you did gain valuable experience and knowledge from your initial run, the first time through something difficult or complicated can actually be easier, precisely because you don't know what's going to happen.

During your first program, everything was exciting—even the hard parts, like figuring out what to eat at a restaurant or dealing with a family dinner. (And when you did figure it out, wasn't it exhilarating?) You had no

* According to a 2015 survey of more than 1,900 Whole30ers

idea what to expect from one day to the next, which meant each morning unfolded like an adventure. Yay, reset!

Okay, maybe not *every* day was magical, but there's something to be said for going through an experience, looking back, and saying, "Whoa, that was really hard . . . but I did it!" Then, when the time comes for you to head into your second round, you already know the hard parts, the parts where you'll struggle, the parts where you'll be frustrated and cranky. (Plus, you know how much work it is, compared to grabbing something healthy but not quite reset-worthy at the deli for lunch.) All these things make the next reset far less appealing, which makes it harder to see the full program all the way through.

If this is your context, make a plan for the tough parts you know are coming. If late nights at the office, travel days, or family dinners were difficult in your first go-round, figure out how you'll handle those your second time through, in order to reduce stress and give yourself a "cushion" for when you're tempted to quit. Also, inject some fun or newness into your second program. Commit to trying two new dinner recipes a week; pair up with a reset "buddy" on social media or your healthy-living forum; or grab lunch at that new place you've been dying to try, and figure out how to stick to the reset on the fly.

LACK OF PREPARATION. If you had a relatively easy time settling into the groove of your first reset, and if you've retained your meal prep skills and kitchen confidence, you may enter into this second reset with a pretty relaxed attitude. You may be thinking, "I've been living in the food freedom zip code for a while now—I've totally got this." The risk is that you may be lulled into a false sense of security. As a result, you won't clean out your pantry, reinstate a support system, plan any meals, or make "if/then" plans for potentially stressful situations.

Because, you know, you got this.

Until two days into your reset, at which point you become acutely aware that you don't, in fact, got this. The food-freedom-appropriate-but-not-reset-worthy convenience foods you've been relying on? Out. That whey-based post-workout shake you've reincorporated? Out. Not sweating whether there's added sugar in your salad dressing? Out. And all of a sudden, you're panicking, because this is harder than you remember, you didn't give it the attention it deserved, and now you're scrambling.

This is easy to prevent. Just remember that *every* reset requires planning and preparation. Go back to page 55 and check off the to-do items.

Um, that's it. Moving on.

FRUSTRATION WITH THE TECHNICALITIES. During your first reset, you were probably very careful about making sure absolutely everything you ate was compliant, because you took the idea of "No cheats, no slips, no excuses" seriously. In addition, you really didn't know what would happen if you got two weeks into the program and accidentally ate soy sauce or peanut butter, and you really didn't want to take the chance of ruining your reset.

Now you're a lot more aware. You think peanut butter isn't a big deal, the cream in your coffee doesn't impact you much (if at all), and a little soy snuck into your sushi is NBD for your body. This makes it much harder to stick to the reset rules, because at this point, you figure, "Meh, I know how XYZ food affects me anyway."

This is dangerous.

This puts you in the mind-set of, "Do I really have to worry about all these other rules, too?" And failing to fully commit to *every* aspect of the reset makes it so much easier to abandon the program when it becomes inconvenient or unpleasant.

Please don't do this.

Every reset is another opportunity to learn even more about how food affects you physically, psychologically, and emotionally. This is the very foundation of your food freedom; making conscious, deliberate decisions based on this information. What you think is just fine/worth it/no problem right now may, in fact, be not so fine/not worth it/actually kind of problematic from one reset to the next. Each reset builds on the last, and brings a greater range and depth of awareness when you reintroduce.

Commit to treating every program like it's your first, from elimination all the way through reintroduction, because it kind of *is* like starting all over again.

A ROUGH RIDE. If you had great success with your first reset but have gone pretty far off the rails (or waited a long time before admitting you needed help), you may think a return to your reset will be nothing but sunshine and rainbows, like a tearful reunion with a childhood friend. And you may be very unpleasantly surprised when the first ten days of your second program are more like a name-calling, hair-pulling, drink-throwing reunion episode of that reality TV show you won't actually admit to watching but secretly love.

Think season 2 of *Vanderpump Rules*. Not that I've seen it.

What I'm trying to say is that your second reset could be just as rough as your first. Perhaps even worse, because you now know how good you *can* feel … and this ain't it. Your Sugar Dragon might roar. Your headaches might return. You might find it hard to crawl out of bed on Day 3, and even harder to face your cheerful co-workers for the morning meeting on Day 6. If you're not prepared for this, it might prove such a shock that you abandon your second attempt altogether.

If you know you're coming back to your reset after a few weeks (or months) of less-than-stellar habits, brace yourself. Return to your reset journal (you kept one, right?), or simply remind yourself of some of the not-so-pleasant moments. Accept that the more immune triggers in your diet before you start your second round, the longer it will take to get you back to feeling awesome. Approach it one week, one day, one meal at a time if you have to. And create a good support network and "if/then" plans up front, so when the going gets tough, you have plenty of options besides bailing.

NO MORE LOW-HANGING FRUIT. Because your first reset was an eye-opening experience and a departure from your past diet and lifestyle, you probably saw dramatic results really fast. But if you've retained most of your new, healthy habits for much of the time since then, your next reset isn't actually the same radical departure. Which means you won't get the same radical results, either.

If you get partway through your second reset and feel better-ish, look better-ish, but get discouraged because you're not seeing the "miracles" or weight loss you saw during the first round, you may be tempted to quit ... and that experience of starting and giving up makes it all the harder to start again.

So, before you reset again, it's time to get real: You probably won't get the same stunning results the second time through, because the reset isn't as drastic of a change, and you've already made so much progress in how you look and feel. (This is especially true of weight loss, which almost always happens fastest in the first stages of a healthy eating effort.) Combat this sense of disappointment by focusing on something different for this reset. Create goals centered around non-scale victories—things that speak to your self-confidence, other health efforts, cooking competence, or socialization And embrace that your second reset can be equally as rewarding as the first, even if you don't lose as much weight or experience a huge burst of energy—if for no other reason than the self-confidence you've gained by seeing it through.

Every Reset Is Different

Whether your second (or third, or fifth) reset is easier or harder than the last, one thing is for certain: It will be different. With every experience, you'll be drawn to other aspects, learn new things, and get more into the nuances of how the elimination and reintroduction of your reset foods impacts you physically, mentally, and emotionally.

SPARE SOME CHANGE?

liken this experience to learning how to drive a car with a dollar bill in your pocket. Say every time you get in a car, you've got $1.00 worth of attention to spend. When you first learn how to drive, you're spending $0.90 on the very act of driving. Seat belt fastened, rearview mirror adjusted, foot on the brake, emergency brake off, check behind, check to the side, check behind again . . . You're spending cents like crazy, and you haven't even left the driveway. As you get more comfortable with driving, however, you're spending less attention on the technical aspects of driving, which leaves you more attention for other things. You notice the beautiful mountains around you, find your favorite song on the radio, and hear that funny whining noise coming from the engine that no one else would notice, but you do, because it's your car. That's how it's going to be with your reset.

In the beginning, you're only going to notice the big things, in part because the changes will be big, and in part because your focus automatically goes to the practical. The first round generally brings huge awareness of the physical impact of your food choices, so you'll feel almost hyper-aware of what's happening with your energy, sleep, digestion, skin, chronic pain, inflammation, and waistline. Through the process, you may also realize you've got emotional ties to and cravings around specific foods and/or circumstances. (Telling your temper-tantrum-throwing brain "no" for the first time in a long time is a pretty big eye-opener.)

Understandably, these may be the only things you notice during the first round of your reset. The changes are huge! You feel totally different! It's like you're driving effortlessly for the first time in your life—and boy, is that worth paying attention to.

After a period of time spent enjoying your food freedom and practicing your "worth it" skills, you'll have even more awareness money to spend. The reset rules, handling food emergencies and social situations, and your general meal prep routine feel familiar, almost habitual. And because your bodily changes probably won't be as dramatic, I'm advising you now to specifically look for other differences before and after your next reset.

You will find *EVEN MORE MAGIC.*

Every experience will bring even more awareness of how food affects you. You'll dive deeper into the nuances of your emotional relationship with food, notice even more subtle effects of giving things up and reintroducing them, and fine-tune your definition of "worth it." To go back to the car analogy, after a few resets, you'll finally be able to hear that tiny little whine that could be the first sign of trouble on the horizon—something you couldn't possibly do during your very first drive.

For me, this was recognizing the subtle effect eating gluten regularly was having on me, which only came to light after my fourth Whole30. I knew from my first (and second, and third) experience that gluten made me bloated, but I never realized what it was doing to my attitude . . . until my fourth reset. After reintroducing gluten a few times on the given day, I realized something: I was cranky. And kind of depressed. In fact, everything sucked, and what was the point, and I might as well just start eating bread again.

It was subtle, but it impacted my mood, my motivation, and my emotional energy. But I had never noticed it before because I was so focused on my belly looking puffy and patiently waiting for any ensuing digestive issues. They never came . . . but as I eventually discovered, that doesn't mean I was totally in the clear when it comes to bread. Or waffles. Or my beloved cupcakes.

These discoveries may not be as fulfilling as the initial "Holy crap, *that's* what's been making my skin break out!" revelations, but they're seriously important. Every piece of information you gather about your relationship with food gets you closer and closer to food freedom. It's how you make better "worth it" decisions. It's how you plan for (or around) the inclusion of certain foods in your life. It means you won't be caught off guard after a few days of croissants in Paris with virtually no physical effects, then coming home and wondering why you can't find the motivation to get back to the gym. For me, it was understanding that I can eat one cupcake and be totally in the clear, but if I eat two, I'll pay the psychological price for the next 36 hours.

Additional information about how many cupcakes I can get away with is critically important to my food freedom. Which brings me to my final point on why subsequent resets are so important to your Food Freedom plan:

Your definition of "worth it" is always changing.

Or at least, it should be. And without challenging your current beliefs, how will you know to adjust your plan to make it work even better for you?

As you continue down this food freedom path, you'll feel like you're effortlessly cycling through one big positive-feedback loop. You'll feel better, so you'll want to do more healthy stuff. Which makes you feel better, which means you'll want to do even more healthy stuff. It's the exact opposite of the cycle you used to be stuck in (where you felt like crap, so you ate more crap, which made you feel even more craptastic).

As you cycle happily through this positive loop, your context is shifting with every step. Your body is changing. Your self-confidence is better. Your energy is more stable. Your entire life is adjusting. That means your goals, health, and tolerance for dietary shenanigans are always changing, too. It's not unusual for something to be deemed "totally worth it" after your first reset, but not actually worth it after your third. Conversely, something may be not worth it now because it physically messes you up, but after a year of gut healing and immunity boosting, you find you can enjoy it periodically without major consequences—it's worth it again!

Each and every reset allows you to refine your definition of "worth it," given how *that* food feels in *that* moment to your *current* body and brain. And even small adjustments to your regular daily diet based on what you've discovered during another reset can make a big difference in how good you look and feel, and how secure you are in your food freedom.

Food Freedom Awaits

And with that, I conclude your three-part Food Freedom plan.

Congratulations! Improved health, changed habits, and an improved relationship with food is just over the horizon. For the first time, you've got a dietary plan that's specifically tailored for you; strategies for successfully managing cravings, stress, and all the curve balls life could throw at you; and a foolproof backup if you ever find yourself off course. You've got it all covered.

FREEDOM!

Until you go to brunch with your best friends. Or dinner at your mom's. Or a business lunch with your closest colleagues.

And then all hell breaks loose.

This could happen. I want to prepare you. So let's talk about how to talk to friends, family, and co-workers about your new healthy-eating plan in a way that won't get you divorced, unfriended, or fired.

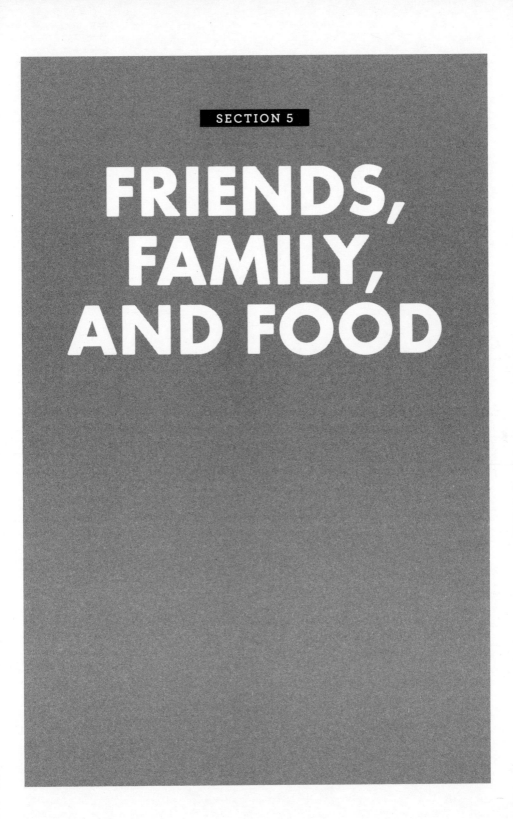

FRIENDS, FAMILY, AND FOOD

CHAPTER 11

TALKING ABOUT YOUR RESET

Taking on a reset is a challenging process. What should you bring to the office potluck? What can you order at your favorite breakfast spot? What kind of snacks should you smuggle onto the airplane? (Answer: all the meat sticks.) But it's more than just your food choices that pose a challenge; you probably didn't anticipate the extent to which your social interactions would change, too. You're not just ordering sparkling water during happy hour—you're fielding questions about why you're not drinking, dealing with peer pressure to have "just one," and wondering if your boss no longer considers you a team player.

Don't underestimate the impact your reset and Food Freedom plan will have on your relationships. While you might assume that family and friends will support you unconditionally, only wanting the best for your health and happiness, that doesn't always happen. A critical notion to keep in mind as you read the next three chapters:

Food isn't just food.

In our relationships, food is love, acceptance, bonding, and comfort. It's a shared indulgence, a way to let off steam, a guilty pleasure made less guilty by the participation of others. Food is sometimes the only way you can connect with certain people in your life. Food is emotional—far more emotional than exercise, meditation, or other activities you may take on to improve your health. With some people, food can be just as sensitive and polarizing a subject as politics or religion.

And you're over here like, "I just asked the waiter to hold the bun?"

Changing the food you put on your plate can make others feel threatened, insulted, uncomfortable, or rejected. Some people will feel guilty just watching you make healthier choices for yourself, even if you do so quietly and without fanfare. And sometimes your efforts to reassure them or defend your choices only make the situation worse. You may be misunderstood. You may be teased. You may be excluded. You may be challenged, peer pressured, or guilt-tripped. This may take place over the course of one lunch, or every single time you find yourself around these people when food is involved. Their pushback can escalate, with jabs changing from passive-aggressive to just plain aggressive. The kitchen table may feel like a battle zone.

The worst part is that your "opponent" is your best friend, boss, or spouse.

If you're caught off guard, these interactions can leave you feeling confused, angry, defensive, or rejected—so much so that you may be tempted to abandon your healthy-eating efforts just to keep the peace. The good news is that you don't have to choose between food freedom and your relationships. There is a way to talk about your new, healthy habits in a way that brings you and the people you love closer together, not further apart.

It's all in the messaging.

Phase 1: Have a Positive Interaction

The first opportunity you'll have to speak to friends and family about your new Food Freedom plan is during your reset, which is both good and bad. It's good because you'll be able to get key "personnel" on board right away, securing their support for the remainder of your reset. It's bad because the elimination is the most restrictive part of this entire process, and if you don't explain it carefully, to the uninitiated, it may sound a little extreme. And by "a little extreme" I mean "crazytownbananapants."

You will, however, approach this carefully.

Ideally, you'll have these conversations ahead of time—*before* Day 1, when you become occupied with the details of the elimination phase itself. (Days 1–10 will be hard enough without having to explain your new "diet" to everyone and their mother.) To set the stage, find a relaxed time to chat with someone, or even a few people all at once. Don't do it at the dinner table or in the kitchen; have the conversation away from food. You wouldn't bring up a touchy sexy-time issue while in bed, would you? Same here: Food is the hot-button issue, and you want to have this conversation on neutral ground. Tell them you'd like to talk to them about a new health effort you'll be starting soon, because you'd really like their support. This can be totally casual: "Hey, I'm going to start this new thing I'm pretty excited about, can I tell you about it?" From here, there are a few directions you could take.

Option 1, which I call the "Shock and Awe," goes something like this: "Starting tomorrow, I'm not eating any grains, dairy, sugar, or junk food. Oh, and I'm not drinking anymore. Turns out, that stuff is really bad for you, and I'm all about eating healthy now."

Yeah, don't do that.

First, this person watched you eat pizza and drink beer just last night, so you're going to come off as ~~kind of~~ wicked hypocritical. Second, this approach immediately puts people on the defensive, because there is a 99.97 percent chance they are consuming at least some of those things in their current diet, and you just took a not-so-subtle dig at their behaviors. Third, it just sounds snotty; no one wants to hang out with the person wearing a "HELLO I'm PREACHY McJUDGERSON" nametag. Seventeenth (this is a *that* bad of an approach), how many times have these people heard you declare, "I'm never drinking again," "I'm really going to clean up my diet (after I crush this bag of kettle chips)," or "That's it, I'm going back to the gym?" That's right: a lot. Sweeping proclamations of a grand nature won't be taken seriously, and are more likely to provoke eye-rolling than cries of support.

Option 2, in which you take a more matter-of-fact angle: "I'm starting a new diet I read about in *Food Freedom Forever*. For thirty days, I'm not allowed to eat any grains, dairy, sugar, junk food, or alcohol, and it's really strict."

Also do not do this. When it comes to your reset, those things are all technically true, but what impact does your language have here? "New diet," "not allowed," and "really strict" make it sound like you're taking on the latest crazy fad diet, blindly following someone else's rules, probably for weight loss. It sounds extreme, it sounds demanding, and to be honest, it sounds like every other diet you've ever gotten excited about in the past. Which means your friends will automatically interpret your words as, "Hey, for the next month, I'm going to be totally obsessive, hungry, cranky, and probably no fun at all."

This is not what you're going for, either.

Here's how Option 3 might sound: "I've been struggling with cravings and energy lately, plus I haven't been sleeping well, which is why I'm drinking All the Coffee. I found this lifestyle program that focuses on changing your habits and your relationship with food, and it makes so much sense to me. I'm going to see if I can use it to break my yo-yo diet cycle, get my cravings in check, and have better energy with less caffeine. I'll be eating way more fruit and vegetables, replacing my nightly wine ritual with something that doesn't mess up my sleep so much, and hopefully learning how to stop shoving chocolate in my mouth every time I'm stressed, because that makes me feel awful about myself."

Now, *that's* a good opener.

It focuses on the many healthy behaviors you will be adopting, and not a laundry list of "don'ts." It emphasizes your long-term goals, all of which are centered on improving your well-being instead of weight loss. And it allows you to share your personal reasons for taking it on, in an open and authentic way that brings you and the other person closer together. In summary, this conversation gets them in your corner, instead of pitting you against each other.

When you have this conversation, try to make your food freedom motivation relatable. Let's say you're talking to a sedentary friend. She won't understand why slower-than-usual workout recovery times or slogging through your 5K is a bummer for you, so pick something she *can* relate to. Share your issues with cravings, poor sleep, allergies, or joint pain—anything that you know she also struggles with, or something that she's watched you battle in the past.

You also want to make your story as personal as is appropriate for your relationship with that person. I'm not suggesting you get into the gory details of your digestive issues with your boss, but don't be afraid to share from the heart with people you're close to. Maybe even let yourself be a little vulnerable. Saying, "I hear this program is good for cravings" isn't anywhere near as powerful as saying, "I'm eating so much junk food, and I just can't stop. It's making me feel like crap about myself. This program tackles cravings head-on, and my self-esteem is ready for a change."

DON'T YOU AGREE?

You may be thinking, "But that's not REALLY what I'm doing—there *is* a pretty serious elimination phase, and I *can't* have pizza or beer, and I should just vomit out all the rules right this minute so they're not surprised tomorrow." Deep breath, baby, and slow your roll. Yes, there is more to share, but your sole goal right now is to have a positive initial interaction, so just start there. Open the conversation as described, then sit back and see how they respond. The beauty of this approach is that it's unlikely to provoke a negative response. No one will say your cravings or energy struggles are fake. Nobody will think breaking the yo-yo diet cycle is a terrible idea. And who would look down on eating more vegetables? That means that all you're going to get out of this conversation is a bunch of head nods, which brings to mind an old sales trick: Get them agreeing with you up front, so when you try to sell them the hard stuff, they're already in the mind-set of saying yes. It's a tiny bit sneaky, but it's for a good cause.

This initial interaction might end here. Your conversation partners may just say, "That sounds great, let me know how it goes," at which point you're done. If they don't ask for more information, don't force it on them. Remember, food is highly emotional, and you've just shared some pretty personal stuff. There is a good chance that what you've said resonated with them. Maybe they're revisiting their own struggles, or questioning their own choices. If that's the case, they may not be ready to hear more about the plan. Or maybe they're happy with (or addicted to) what they're doing and thinking, "Lovely that you're trying to drink less coffee, but I will kick your shin if you tell *me* to cut back." Regardless, when it comes to food, let them come to you. If they want to know more about the plan, they'll ask.

If your initial conversation does prompt follow-up questions, answer them, but stick to the plan: Keep it positive, avoid buzzwords (like "diet" or "cleanse") that may have a negative connotation, and make it personal and relatable. They'll likely ask for more information about the program, like what it's called, how it works, or specifically what you'll be eating. Here's how your answers might sound, based on a variety of potential inquiries. (Fill in your own specifics related to your motivations and goals.)

THEM: "Tell me more about this plan."

YOU: "It's from a book called *Food Freedom Forever*. The program helps you identify food sensitivities, change bad habits, and pinpoint emotional attachments to foods. It's not about eating perfectly or never drinking wine again; it's going to teach me how the foods I've been eating are affecting me and how to enjoy things like my mom's chocolate-chip cookies with a sense of control and without guilt."

THEM: "So it's a diet."

YOU: "It's not actually a diet, in the way most people think about diets. The goal isn't weight loss; it's a complete reboot of my health, habits, and relationship with food. There is no calorie counting or points, and there are no pills, powders, or shakes—I'll just be eating real food, as much as my body needs. I've even committed to not stepping on the scale for the next month, so I can really focus on changing my habits and observing what happens to my energy, sleep, mood, digestion, and athletic performance. I need to break my scale addiction anyway, and I'm looking forward to getting back in touch with how good it feels to eat healthy without worrying about whether I'm losing weight."

THEM: "How does it work?"

YOU: "Part of the program is identifying foods that aren't working well for me—things that may be promoting cravings, screwing up my metabolism, upsetting my digestion, or disrupting my immune system and creating symptoms. I'm using it to figure out what's been making my skin break out and my belly bloat. There's an elimination phase, where I leave out commonly problematic foods, and a reintroduction phase, where I bring them back in and see how they work for me. After that, I get to decide whether I want them in my everyday diet or not based on my experience."

THEM: "What's your goal?"

YOU: "For the next month, I'm committing to eating nothing but healthy protein; tons of vegetables and fruit; and natural fats. I'm going to stick to it 100%, so when I reintroduce the foods I've been leaving out at the end of the month, I can really evaluate the difference—how I felt without them, and how I feel with them. This will be a great learning experience. When it's over, I'll know exactly how certain foods have been contributing to my cravings, allergies, even my shoulder pain, and I'll have all the information necessary to create the perfect diet for me."

THEM: "What do you eat?"

YOU: "I'll be eating nutritious foods with protein, healthy fats, and fiber, which will keep me satisfied and help me trust the 'hungry' and 'full' signals my body is sending me. I'll be eating way more vegetables, too. Because I won't be eating the stuff I usually pig out on when I'm anxious or lonely, I'll have space to get in touch with my feelings and can learn to comfort myself in a healthy way. I'm using the program to help me gain control of food again, because the last few months of emotional eating and guilt have been really hard, and I haven't been able to break the cycle on my own."

All of these responses are designed to bring you and your conversation partners closer together, by sharing the positive aspects of the program and your personal reasons for taking it on. Notice one thing you're NOT doing: Providing a laundry list of all of the foods you *won't* be eating for the next 30 days. The tendency is to jump straight to the rules, but if you did that first, all you'd hear is how crazy or extreme it sounds—or your plan would be written off as just another weight-loss fad diet. Once your friends understand why you're doing this and how important it is to you, the efforts you'll be going through to achieve your health goals won't sound so extreme.

TIMING IS EVERYTHING

Don't bring up how "strict" or "extreme" the reset phase is, how hard it will be, or how the first week or two are probably going to suck. Yes, that does fall under "sharing your authentic thoughts," but now isn't the time to be quite so authentic. Share the tough stuff *after* they agree that this is a worthy pursuit and have agreed to support you in your efforts; start talking about that now and you'll only plant the idea that you're setting yourself up for failure.

Now, imagine you've had these discussions exactly the way I've outlined them. Chances are, you've achieved your goal of a positive interaction, and your friends, family, or co-workers are nodding their heads right along with you. So far, so good. Then, they ask you about the rules: "So what, specifically, are you not eating?"

Before you blurt out your reset "no" list, pause.

There's a trick I use when a member of the media asks me a question I don't really want to answer, or approaches a topic I *do* want to talk about from a negative or biased angle: I simply answer the question I *wanted* them to ask, staying mostly on topic without falling into any potential traps and making sure I get my messaging across. You can channel this here.

First, lead with what you *are* eating, even if they asked what you're leaving out. In the case of a Whole30 reset, you'd say, "I'm eating meat, seafood, and eggs; lots of vegetables and fruit; and healthy fats. Think pan-seared salmon and poached eggs drizzled in hollandaise with a side of fresh berries; warm chicken salad with roasted butternut squash, chopped pecans, diced apple, and a homemade balsamic dressing; and a bison burger topped with a fried egg, caramelized onions, and garlic aioli in a roasted eggplant 'bun.'" (Give them straight-up food porn here, because literally zero persons will hear this list and think, "OMG that sounds AWFUL.")

THE ELEVATOR PITCH

You'll probably get questions about what you're eating a LOT. If you waffle, stammer, or ramble on in your response, they're likely to think you're unclear about the plan, not particularly committed, or already expecting a negative response. It would be helpful to develop an "elevator pitch" here—a short, succinct summary of the plan designed to help you "sell" it to your conversation partner. A good template: "I'm eating X, Y, and Z for the next # days. It looks like ABC Sample Meal. I'm hoping to achieve goals 1, 2, and 3." Keep it positive, keep it simple, and then *practice*. Refine it as you get feedback, or stick with what's working. The more confident you sound in describing the plan, the more it will seem like you're totally in charge and committed to the process.

Then, just wait. Let them react. This may be the end of that—or they may still follow up with, "So what's on your no list, again?"

Now, you're going to answer. The goal isn't to ditch the question forever, just to set them up with a really positive outlook on what you'll be doing first. By now you've had ten-plus minutes of positive conversation, setting you up perfectly to talk about the hard part—what you're leaving out.

Use caution here, too. Keep it simple. Don't be overly dramatic. Most important, don't get defensive before they even comment.

"On the first part of the reset, I won't be eating any grains, legumes, or dairy. I'm also avoiding added sugar, and I won't be drinking for a month."

Then, just wait. Let them react, because they may surprise you. After all this discussion, they might just say, "So it's kind of like Paleo?" or "Well, that sounds tough, but it's for a good cause." Or maybe, if you've sold it well enough: "Interesting. I might want to try this too."

If they start talking about how crazy it is, how restrictive it seems, or ask how anyone can even survive without the Grain food group (I'm sorry, what?), stay calm, acknowledge their fears, and counter gently.

> **YOU:** "It sounds like a lot, but remember, it's only 30 days. After the reset, I'll bring those foods back into my diet to see how they impact me."
>
> "I'm just eating whole, real, nutritious food for a month. I'll finally learn how to cook, too. I bet grandma would say this is the way she used to eat!"
>
> "It did sound restrictive at first, but when I looked at all the delicious food I get to eat and know that I don't have to count calories to succeed, it actually sounded pretty awesome."
>
> "No alcohol for a month, gah, I know, but I can't wait to see how it impacts my sleep and cravings, and I bet I'll work out more too. I'm up for the challenge."

Keep this part short; now isn't the time to get into a heated back-and-forth if they continue to badmouth the plan. If, despite your best efforts, you just can't find common ground at this stage, call a time-out. Thank them for listening and sharing their thoughts. Tell them you'll think about what they said, and would love to talk about it more later. Give everyone some time to cool off, because if their reaction is that extreme, there is probably something emotional at the root. Then, skip ahead to page 197 and read the "dealing with pushback" tactics before your next interactions.

If they still seem agreeable or you are able to overcome their objections after another conversation, it's time to move you both into Phase 2.

Phase 2: Ask for Their Support

Phase 2 is all about marshalling some support during your reset.

What's that? You think that just because they love you, their support is a done deal?

That's so cute.

But not quite.

From their perspective, all you've done so far is share information. "Here's what I'm doing, here's what it will look like, here's what I hope to accomplish." Nowhere in there have you mentioned what you'll need from them throughout the process—or that you even *do* need anything from them. So don't be surprised if all they say here is, "Okay, cool, good luck," and move right on.

General life lesson: People aren't mind-readers.

If you need support, you'll have to ask.

Social support, especially in-person help from those you spend the most time with, will be mission-critical to your food freedom success—a message echoed by nearly everyone who has ever done a Whole30. As Stephanie D. explained on her blog, "I felt nervous to tell people that I was doing the reset. I wasn't confident that I had the willpower to see it through, and I was terrified that people would be watching, expecting me to fail or give up. But I'm so glad I decided to share my plan publicly. My family and friends have been really supportive. Friends messaged me to see how it was going, and I felt proud every time I was able to say I was staying on track. Announcing my participation actually kept me from being tempted to slip or cheat, because I knew people were rooting for me. I won't say that I couldn't have done it without them, but it would have been infinitely more difficult."

In order to garner that type of response, you have to have the conversation. This could go a few ways.

Option 1 is a simple, "Will you support me?" On the plus side, you'll probably get a yes, because no one wants to be the jerk who says, "No way, you're on your own here." But at this point, neither of you knows what "supporting" really means, so the request (and the affirmative response) are virtually meaningless. Will this person support you by bullying you into completing the reset at all costs, or by being sympathetic if you tell her you want to quit? Is the occasional high-five going to do the trick, or do you need some daily one-on-one time to talk about how you're actually feeling? Are they supposed to ask you how it's going, or will the constant check-ins be annoying?

You need to have a more in-depth conversation.

Option 2: In an attempt at camaraderie, you might try to recruit them as a major player in your reset. "I need you to hold me to this. Make sure I stick to it!" or "Promise you'll make sure I finish this—I've failed at diets too often, and I don't want to fail here, too."

While your intentions are good, and they might love the blood-brothers-we're-in-this-together-you-are-my-person vibe, this can only end badly.

You're trying to get them on your team, but this approach puts them in a can't-win position. Let's illustrate with a story: You're on this new diet, and you're supposed to avoid all sweets. You tell your co-worker, "No candy for me. If you see my hand in the candy jar, slap it!" Your co-worker fist-bumps you in agreement—she's got your back!

You stick to your guns for a while, but eventually, something happens (a tough day, a missed lunch, a late meeting, you've been *so good* . . .), and you find yourself reaching for the communal jar of mini-Snickers. Your co-worker notices and cheerfully says, "Hey, you said no candy!" And what do you snap back with?

"Look, *Pam*, I am a *grown-up person*, and if I want to eat candy, I can eat candy. It's been a long day and I've been really good and it's just one freakin' Snickers, and it's MINI, so it's FINE."

Well, that's awkward.

Putting someone else in this no-win position never goes well; either they'll do their job and you'll resent them for it, or you won't *let* them do their job, and they'll feel frustrated. This approach also makes you feel like you can relax on your resolve because you have someone else to keep you in line if you feel like slipping. Which isn't real, because the only person who can do this for you is *you*.

Your Option 3 strategy (the good one) is three-fold: Remind them of your personal reasons for taking this on; ask them for what you need, specifically; and tell them how this will benefit your relationship, because everyone wants to know what's in it for them. It could sound like this:

TALKING TO YOUR TEENAGE CHILDREN: "I really want to stick with this plan because I'll have more energy, and it will help me sleep better. I'd love to actually stay awake during our movie nights, and I know I've been cranky and tired after work most days. This plan means I'll be cooking way more, and we won't be ordering out for pizza as much, so please, no whining about that. I'll also need you to move your cookies and chips to a different cabinet, because if I see them every day, it'll be harder for me to resist. Will you help me out on this?"

TALKING TO YOUR SIGNIFICANT OTHER: "My cravings are out of control, and it's really hurting my self-confidence. I want to be able to enjoy dessert with you without beating myself up about it for hours—we'll both enjoy Date Night so much more if I can do that. But my cravings might be intense, so please don't offer me candy or wine, even if you're joking. It may be hard to say no, and I really want to see this through. Can you work with me on that?"

TALKING TO YOUR CO-WORKERS: "I'm dying with allergy season right now, and I'm pretty sure stuff I'm eating is making them worse. If I can figure that out, I'll be more alert during the day, and I'll be way more productive in the afternoon, which will make our whole team happy. I'll still be at every Friday happy hour because I'll definitely need to vent about this project we're working on, but no peer pressure to drink, okay? I promise I'll be just as fun, but I really need to eliminate alcohol to see how that's impacting my symptoms. Cool?"

TALKING TO YOUR BEST FRIENDS: "I'm dragging these days—my energy sucks, I'm not getting any stronger in the gym, and some days it's hard to even get up to work out. I think this new nutrition program is going to help me sleep better, recover faster, and get stronger. It'll be tough to pass on beer and pizza, but I have to commit 100% to this or I won't be able to tell if it's really working. Just leave my sparkling water and salad alone, and I won't rub it in your face when I'm kicking your butts in the gym. Deal?"

Notice something all three scenarios have in common? The very last sentence, where you specifically ask them to buy in. You're looking for another "yes" here—a commitment to either helping you through this or, at the very least, not messing with you during the process. You'll want to tailor the conversation to your subjects, your goals, and the challenges you anticipate, but that final, "You in this with me?" will help you seal the deal.

Recognize, too, that you'll want different forms of support from different people, and be strategic about how you "assign" support jobs. Ask your best friend for tough love, your mom for unconditional praise ("You're doing great, keep it up!"), and your kitchen-whiz co-workers for recommendations when you're struggling with meal boredom. Keep in mind the strengths and personalities of each member of your support team, and only ask for something you know they'll be comfortable giving you. (Your new administrative assistant is likely *not* the right person to ask for tough love.)

DON'T SKIP OUT

Make sure everyone knows you won't be backing out of family traditions, workplace events, or friendly get-togethers just because you're eating a little differently. You'll undermine these conversations entirely if you tell your kids, "Sorry, I can't do movie night, Daddy's not eating popcorn right now." Explain that your relationships aren't dependent on the food you put on your plate (or the drinks in your glass), then walk the talk by continuing to show up to book club, family night, or Sunday brunch with the girls. You promised that your healthy eating efforts would bring you closer together, so demonstrate how that's true by preserving these rituals and bellying up to the bar with your co-workers (and ordering your sparkling water and lime with confidence).

Significant Others

Conversations with your significant other are important enough to warrant their own section, especially if you find the one person who means the most isn't reacting to these conversations the way you hoped they would. Your husband, partner, girlfriend, etc., may be skeptical about your chances of success, negative about the whole idea, or annoyed that you're shaking up your lives in such a dramatic fashion.

Success in this situation can be hard. This is the person with whom you spend the most time and rely on the most for support. You cook together and eat together. You stock the same pantry and refrigerator. You share rituals, traditions, and habits. Their disapproval, apathy, or resistance has serious potential to impact your commitment and motivation. Dealing with unsupportive significant others requires a careful strategy designed to get you back on the same team—or at the very least, keep you feeling strong enough to honor your commitment.

Assuming you've already had the initial conversations (what you'll be doing, why you're doing it, and what you hope to accomplish), the next step is setting expectations. It's possible that a practical discussion about how your reset plans will affect your partner will be enough to relieve his or her concerns.

Have you said, "I don't expect you to do it, too"?

That alone may be what's holding your loved one back from being supportive. Your boyfriend is visualizing you dumping out all his beer; your wife is worried you'll be proclaiming the living room a carb-free zone; your husband is wondering whether Steve's wife is cool with him crashing on the couch in their reset-free living room. For, like, a month.

Have this conversation during a time when you're both relaxed, and away from food. Go for a walk, sit down after work when you're both winding down, or find 15 minutes while the kids are playing to have a conversation. Again, do not do this at the dinner table. (For sake of ease, I'm using "his" from now on, but these conversations work exactly the same with your girlfriend or wife.)

Explain that this effort is yours and yours alone, and you have zero expectations that your partner will do it with you. Promise not to harass him for anything he eats or drinks, reassure him you won't be throwing out his food, and swear you won't rub your amazing energy, glowing skin, and flatter stomach in his face. Much.

Maybe just say that last part to yourself.

Then, invite your S.O. to help you map out your food storage, grocery shopping, and mealtime strategy together. (This is especially important if you're the primary shopper/meal planner/chef.) But before you barge in with all kinds of directives, ask him how he'd like to handle these things. "What could we do to make this a good experience for you, too? Let's brainstorm together." (The idea of "we" is important—you want to remind him that even though you're embarking on this new food adventure solo, you're still a team in all other areas.)

Maybe he'll surprise you here. Maybe, hearing that you're honoring his feelings and not getting defensive, he'll offer to help with meal planning, eat the same dinner as you, or buy his own junk food. That would be cool.

Maybe he won't do that, but he will push the plan back on you. "You're the one who wanted to do this—you tell me." Okaaaay. Take a deep breath, because you can work with this. In this case, you should have some ideas at the ready. Some things to address:

REGARDING JUNK FOOD AND TREATS:

* Where will his junk food go, so you're not tripping over it every time you reach into the pantry?

* Will you pick up treats for him when you grocery shop, or will he have to buy those himself?

- Is it cool if he makes popcorn/drinks wine/orders pizza without warning, or will you ask him to give you a heads-up first?

REGARDING MEAL TIME AND COOKING:

- Does he want to be involved in meal planning, or are you solely in charge?

- Will you cook two totally different meals every night so as not to inconvenience him at all? (Just kidding! This is not a viable option. You know that, right?)

- Will you cook one compliant meal and that's that—"You'll eat what I make and you'll like it"?

- Is he welcome to prepare and add his own pasta/rice/bread as a side?

- When you meal-prep for breakfast and lunch (batch-roasting veggies, grilling chicken breasts, making salad dressing, and hard-boiling eggs), are you making extra for him?

- Does he understand that if he says no and then eats some of your hard-boiled eggs, there will be hell to pay?

You should think about all these things ahead of time and come to the virtual table with an idea of what you will and will not do. Work through these items one by one, compromising where you can and thanking him when and where he compromises, too. Bonus: This will show him you've really thought this through and aren't impulsively jumping on some quick-fix bandwagon wholly unprepared.

Assuming you come to an agreement here, take his temperature again. "I hope that makes you feel better. Can I count on your support this month?" That may be the end of it—yay! If he still has some grumbles, though, it's time to hear him out. Ask him what, specifically, he's worried about. Don't rebut, respond, or deny at this point. Just listen. Give him a minute to share his side of the story, and remember not to take any of his feedback personally. This is not about you; it has everything to do with him. Your job is simply to acknowledge his experience as valid, even if it's not how you see it.

"I know that it sounds like a lot. It is a big change. I hear your concerns that it will be too stressful. I understand you're worried about it messing up your plans. Thank you for sharing all of that. Your feelings are important to me."

DEEP BREATH

It might be *really* tough to keep your cool here, especially if he comes out of the gate pretty aggressively anti-reset ... but you have to. Make sure you're in a good place and feeling generous before you initiate this conversation, because if you retreat into defensiveness, you have no hope of creating a plan that will actually work. He's struggling with something here. This is hard. Find some compassion, take nothing personally, and be the bigger person for the greater good.

Once you acknowledge his feelings, *then* you can work through some of the questions or criticisms he may have, using the strategies I'm about to outline in chapter 12. Perhaps a more thorough explanation of the plan, your goals, and your expectations will help smooth over some of his concerns.

If none of this works, however—if you *still* can't come up with a good plan together and he's *still* having a hard time finding support for you—it's time to fall back. "I'm sorry we can't seem to find anything that works for you here; let's just agree to disagree on the concept for now. I've committed to thirty days of this plan and I'm going to see it through, but I will do my best not to make any part of it difficult for you."

Then, just chill.

This way of eating is likely very new to both of you, and unknowns in a relationship are always a little scary. Accept that this is just how it is, and adjust your support plan accordingly. If you continue to hound him ("Can't you at least ask me how it's going once in a while?"), you'll create distance. If you resent him for not stepping up, you'll create distance. If you tune him out entirely because you're frustrated with his response, you'll create distance. Don't let that happen. Find compassion. Understand that everyone comes to these things in their own time, and in their own way. If you can't expect anything but "No comment" from him in the beginning, so be it. Look to others for support, encouragement, and advice, and let him off the hook, because the last thing you want is food freedom at the expense of your relationship.

There is a good chance if you just let it roll, you'll find your partner's attitude much improved once you both get used to it and he sees how much happier and healthier it's making you.

Care to Join Me?

Throughout these conversations, you may be secretly looking for more than just support—what you'd really like is a reset buddy. You might be angling for someone to take the program on because doing it together would be a great bonding experience. Maybe you've been watching a particular person struggle with his or her health, habits, or relationship with food and believe the program will help. Or, perhaps, because you know you stand a much better chance of actually seeing it through if your spouse/ roommate/parents do it with you. (P.S. You're right: All the studies show that most behavioral changes, from weight loss to quitting smoking, are easier when you have a partner in crime.)

It's okay to be a little bit selfish in your intentions, but the other person has to be the one to bring it up. No, really, they do, for three reasons: One, their health is none of your business, no matter how much you love them. Two, the only person you can effectively be responsible for here is *you*. Three, can you even imagine how you'd recruit them? "Hey, I'm starting this new healthy-eating program, and boy, could you use some of that!" (Let me know how that works out.) Even if you come up with kinder way of extending an invitation, it could still be perceived as judgment or criticism, provoking defensiveness, anger, or hurt feelings.

Talking about food is tricky. Err on the side of caution and wait to see if they come to you.

If they do extend feelers about the program details or express interest in doing it too, respond positively, but keep it casual. No sudden moves; don't startle the wildlife. Try something like:

> **YOU:** "If you want, I can lend you my book so you can read more about it."
>
> "It would be fun to learn how to cook together—check out this amazing recipe I want to try."
>
> "If we can get through the Tough Mudder together, I'm pretty sure we could handle a month of black coffee."

Then just wait. You really need them to come all the way to you; if they feel pushed in any way this early in the process, they may retreat.

STILL THINKING

Psychologists who study the stages of behavioral change call this the "contemplative phase," in which people weigh the pros and cons of changing their behavior. You may feel really excited as you watch your friend or partner enter this phase—"Yes, they're actually going to do this with me!"—but temper your enthusiasm. People can remain in this contemplative stage for months or even years before actually taking action. Be patient, spend more of your time helping them gather information and less time convincing them to get on board, and let your results speak for themselves.

If they continue to pursue the idea, have some plans at the ready. Imagine all the support you'll be able to offer each other through the process, then share your vision with them. Remember to emphasize all the ways this experience will bring you closer together, in addition to the many other benefits.

> **YOU:** "We could plan on dinner at each other's houses once a week and try out new recipes."
>
> "We can batch-cook together on Sunday nights while we catch up on *Grey's Anatomy*."
>
> "We'll be each other's phone-a-friend; any time we have a craving, just text and we'll talk each other down."

You can also ask, "If we did this together, how could I help you through the process? What would you need to feel supported and be successful?"

Then just wait. If you get a reset buddy out of these conversations, awesome! But if they're just not ready, back off. I know they just got you all excited and hopeful, but if they're not ready, *they're not ready.*

Change is hard.

Don't get emotional. Don't beg and plead. And for the love of Bieber, don't drop the hammer in a last-ditch effort to get them on board. Spewing out, "You're twenty pounds overweight, you need three cups of coffee just to wake up, and you're addicted to sugar. Something has to change!" isn't motivating; it's just mean.

If the other person isn't willing to address their less-than-healthy behavior, there is nothing you can do to make it happen. Plus, pushing them here will jeopardize any chance you had of getting them to support you in the first place. Thank them for their interest, acknowledge that talking about this isn't easy, and tell them how grateful you are to have a friend like them. Then hug it out and move on.

Lead by Quiet Example

One last word on the subject of friends, family, and food: When trying to get someone to come around to your new healthy habits, rarely will preaching, guilt-tripping, or stunning displays of logic work. And by "rarely" I mean "not a snowball's chance in hell."

The only tactic that *does* stand a chance (but it's a good chance) is leading by quiet example.

Translation: You do you.

Eat your food. Don't make a big deal out of it. Feel and look amazing. Don't make a big deal out of it. Be insanely proud of yourself. Don't make a big deal out of it. If someone compliments you on your commitment, skin, or waistline, say, "Thanks, I feel great," and then be quiet. Have more energy, better focus, a most positive outlook, and fewer aches and pains, but don't rub it in. Lead by quiet example, and wait to see if they'll come to you.

If they do, answer their questions, but as I've said, don't press them too hard. Make it clear that you're there if and when they're ready, but you're not going to force anything. Based on my Whole30 experience, resistant parties are far more likely to come around when they see your incredible results speaking for themselves.

Until then, however, they may still be kind of bratty about it.

I told you, food is *hard*.

CHAPTER 12

DEALING WITH PUSHBACK

No matter how careful your approach or how much your friends and family want to see you happy, you still might get some pushback on your reset. (And if it doesn't come from them, you might hear it from a casual acquaintance or friend-of-a-friend you encounter while socializing.) No one would take issue with the big-picture goals of changing your health, habits, or relationship with food (because who's gonna say *that* sounds dumb?), but your restaurant order, post-workout meal, or sparkling water at happy hour may draw attention, and the rules and structure of your reset protocol may invite teasing, criticism, or skepticism.

This is understandable. Think about the very first time you read the rules of your reset. Your reaction probably ranged from, "Wow, that's a lot of stuff I can't eat" to "Aw, HELL NO." It's intimidating, and it's probably a little scary for people to imagine, even if they're not doing the program themselves.

That said, please don't assume everyone is going to give you a hard time about your new healthy eating plan. Anticipating their criticism can make you behave defensively, which could prompt family and friends to react to your *behavior*, not the plan itself. (Translation: By anticipating a conflict, you might actually instigate one!) Whole30er Allyson C. knows this firsthand: "In reality, it was pretty easy to talk to friends and family about my reset, but my perception going into these conversations was that it was going to be a battle. I was expecting negative comments, and that created more anxiety than necessary. My expectation of the pushback actually changed my behavior and diverted my focus."

I'm going to give you a wide variety of examples of the kind of criticism you might encounter in this chapter, but that doesn't mean you'll encounter all (or any) of them. I just want you to be prepared in case you do, giving you a way to respond kindly in the heat of the moment. But let's enact one rule of thumb here:

Expect the best.

Don't assume that everyone you eat lunch with is going to make fun of your diet, tempt you with off-plan treats, or criticize what's on your plate. It's far more likely that they'll just be curious, accept what you're doing matter-of-factly, or not even notice you're eating a little differently. You may not need any of the tips in this chapter at all, in fact.

But just in case...

If you do experience criticism, skepticism, or teasing, you'll ideally receive that feedback calmly and with an open mind. Assume the other person is just trying to understand, not bash your decision or the plan. See if you can find truth in the points they are trying to make, then thank them for their concern and respond thoughtfully. Above all, *don't get defensive*. This isn't a personal attack on you; they're just questioning the program.

Let's talk about the most common criticisms you might hear, and how you can handle them gracefully. These are all valid concerns when it comes to your reset, so if you encounter any of these, answer them as calmly, concisely, and helpfully as you can.

"I COULD NEVER DO THAT; I LOVE BREAD TOO MUCH." This isn't a direct criticism, but you still have to handle it carefully. Don't try to suggest they really could or come up with all the reasons why they should at least try. Acknowledge their feelings, and keep your response simple. They're already feeling slightly defensive, so don't say anything that could be perceived as critical of them, like, "It's only thirty days!" Try something like, "I hear you! It's definitely going to be challenging." Or keep it light: "I know, I actually googled, 'hamburger bun replacements'!" And then just leave it alone, because this comment is just an indicator of their own struggles with food.

"THAT DOESN'T SOUND SUSTAINABLE." Remind them that the reset is designed to be a short-term learning experience, not a lifelong set of rules to follow. Tell them that after the 30 days, you're looking forward to reintroducing the foods that you've missed, to see how you might incorporate them back into your healthy lifestyle. If this isn't your first reset, you can bring in specific examples from your own history. "During my first Whole30, I figured out that dairy really upset my stomach, so now I skip cheese unless it's a really special dish. Without that reset, I never would have known what was making my belly bloat. And it turns out avoiding cheese really isn't hard for me, so it's been a major win in terms of my quality of life."

"BUT YOU DON'T NEED TO LOSE WEIGHT." Even if you've clearly explained food freedom as a health- and habit-focused approach, people still equate eating healthier with the desire to slim down. Share your personal reasons for taking on this reset, because it bears repeating: "I'm not doing this for weight loss. I'm truly looking to improve my energy, see if I can figure out what's upsetting my digestion, and get my cravings under control." If they're worried that you can't afford to lose any weight, explain that because there is no calorie restriction, you'll make sure you're eating enough to support your muscle mass and activity levels.

"YOU'LL BE MISSING OUT ON KEY NUTRIENTS." This one often comes from someone who read a magazine article on the "dangers" of eating gluten-free or Paleo. Acknowledge that, yes, grains have fiber and dairy has calcium, but you'll be eating tons of fresh, nutritious food, including lots of vegetables and fruit, and getting a wide variety of vitamins, minerals, and fiber from other healthy sources. You can outline a day of sample meals so they can see how nutritious your reset diet is, or point out that you can get just as much fiber in a half cup of blackberries as two slices of toast. Finally, let them know that your reset is designed to improve your digestion, which means you'll be better able to absorb the vitamins and minerals in your food.

"BUT ALL THOSE THINGS ARE SO HEALTHY!" You may also get specific concerns about cutting out "healthy" foods like low-fat dairy or whole grains. This is where I'll direct you back to page 34, where I talked about these foods not as "good" or "bad," but as "unknown for you." Explain to your conversation partner that there *are* good things in these foods, but they are also commonly problematic, and you just want to find out how they work for you. If you have a specific symptom or issue, cite that. "My allergies are so bad right now, and I'm wondering if something I'm eating is making them worse."

"WHY DOES IT HAVE TO BE SO ALL-OR-NOTHING?" This generally comes from people who believe that willpower or moderation is the answer to any body weight or diet concern. I covered this back on page 27, but you'll want to personalize your response. "If I could eat everything in moderation, I would. But I can't, because certain foods make me feel totally out of control. This short-term reset is going to help me get a better handle on my cravings and relationship with food, so I *will* be able to enjoy those things in moderation later, if I want to." (You can also cite the basics tenets of an elimination diet here, in which the effectiveness depends on 100% compliance during the elimination phase.)

"THERE GOES YOUR SOCIAL LIFE." While you may be intimidated at the idea of navigating a restaurant menu, birthday party, or happy hour while on your reset, don't let 'em see you sweat. "I'm not going to turn into a hermit just because I'm eating healthy, and it's not going to be that hard. I know exactly what I will and won't be eating, I'll do my homework ahead of time, and I won't make a big deal about it if you won't. Besides, social events are about getting together with you guys; it doesn't matter what we're actually eating."

"UNLESS YOU HAVE CELIAC, THERE'S NO NEED TO EAT GLUTEN-FREE." This is a tough one, given some recent mainstream media articles that (erroneously) suggested that gluten sensitivity doesn't exist outside of celiac disease. Don't try to out-science them; instead, keep it personal. "I'm not sure whether gluten is an issue for me, but I know that grains in general are problematic for a lot of people, to varying degrees. This plan will help me figure that out. Plus, I like the extra nutrition I'll be getting by replacing bread and pasta with vegetables and fruit for thirty days."

Finally, with all these concerns, emphasize there is an elimination *and* reintroduction phase. "I'm cutting these foods out as part of the experiment, but I am going to bring them back in to see how they affect me. If it's all good, I can certainly decide to start eating them again."

Say "can" here, not "will." Because there's a very good chance you won't always want to.

QUOTE SCIENCE CAREFULLY

You may be tempted to quote the latest *Science Daily* article or that statistic you read in *It Starts with Food*, but unless biochemistry is your full-time job, steer away from this strategy. First, you can find "science" to back up just about anything you want to prove, which will just provoke a "he said, she said" argument over whether grains truly are heart-healthy. Second, unless you understand all the nuances of the science very well, you're likely to stumble with follow-up questions, reducing your credibility. Finally, even the strongest scientific research simply can't compete with your personal experience. Saying, "In this study, grains created transient permeability in the gut" isn't anywhere near as effective as saying, "When I gave up grains, my shoulder tendinitis went away. When I started eating bread again, it came back. There must be something in grains that makes my shoulder unhappy, so I just don't eat them." Drop mic, walk away.

There's also one bomb-proof, guaranteed-to-work response to all these inquiries, especially if you're talking to a member of your parents' generation: "I actually explained the whole thing to my doctor, and she thinks it's a great program," or "Don't worry, I talked to my doctor about this ahead of time." If you can get your health-care provider on board with the specifics of your reset, it'll be really hard for anyone else to argue with their professional endorsement. (Plus, you should check with your doctor before you start any new diet or lifestyle program anyway—he or she could even help you choose the best reset for you, given your context.) The Whole30 has some great resources for talking to your doctor about doing the program, written by highly-respected functional medicine practitioner Luc Readinger, MD. Visit whole30.com/tag/talk-to-your-doc for details.

Finally, despite your most valiant efforts, your friends and family may still not understand why you need to do this, or may not agree that it's a good idea. If you get to this point and people are just not picking up what you're putting down, fall back. "Well, I appreciate you hearing me out. I still think this is the best thing I could do for my health right now. If you're interested, I can let you know how it goes when my reset and reintroduction are over—otherwise, you won't hear me mention it again."

And then don't. Your best strategy in this situation is just to do your thing calmly and quietly, without drawing any extra attention to the fact that you're eating a little differently these days. Recognize that as much as it stinks, these aren't the people you can count on for support (at least not yet), so find others to lean on. Don't withdraw socially; show them that you're the same family member/friend/co-worker regardless of what's on your plate.

But don't let anyone push you around, either.

As Buddha famously said, "Do no harm, but take no crap."

Just Say No (to Peer Pressure)

"Just have one, it won't kill you."

"But I made them just for you—they're your favorite."

"What, you're too healthy now to enjoy a donut with the rest of us?"

"Uh oh, hide the chips, here comes Mr. Health Nut."

During your reset, you may find yourself in a situation where your social status, commitment to your health, and self-confidence are tested in an ugly way. This is just as likely to come from a total stranger, a colleague, or your own mother, and you need to be prepared—beyond exclaiming, "What the hell, *Becky*, you're supposed to be my best friend."

There are a number of reasons why people might give you a hard time when you change your diet to include healthier fare. Identifying where they're coming from, finding some empathy, and responding without anger or defensiveness can save this exchange of words from turning into a food fight and keep you on track with your healthy-eating plan.

CONCERN FOR YOU. Your family, friends, and co-workers may genuinely be concerned for your health or sanity on this plan, especially if you didn't get the chance to talk to them about the details of the plan up front. They may have witnessed you jumping from diet to diet in the past, getting excited about each new plan, then watching your self-esteem plummet (and your waistline expand) when the latest and greatest just doesn't work long term. It's understandable that they don't want to see you go through that again.

If they're worried about you cutting out whole food groups, becoming obsessed with your body weight, or falling prey to yet another fad diet, educate them on how a reset is different. Emphasize that this isn't a quick fix or a Band-Aid, and it's not about weight loss—you'll be focusing on your habits and emotional relationship with food. Outline a sample day of meals or flash some photos of what you've been eating to show them you're not starving, and the food isn't actually weird.

What do you mean, you haven't been taking pictures of your food? Those baked chicken thighs with creamy tarragon dressing over charred leeks aren't going to Instagram themselves, you know.

They may also feel bad for you because you're missing out on all the fun foods they get to eat. They may assume you feel deprived, are always ravenous, or feel left out when everyone orders a beer and you're drinking water.

Don't lie about this.

If you say, "Oh, no, I would much rather eat a grilled chicken salad than pizza, and I don't even miss beer," it's going to come off as inauthentic, because it's probably not true. So be honest, but reassure them, too.

You're not being waterboarded, you're just drinking your coffee black.

Try saying something like, "You know, I do have cravings, and yes, it's hard when everyone is drinking beer and I have water. But most of the time, I feel really great. I know this is only a short-term experiment, and I'm already feeling more energetic and less bloated, which is really motivating me to stick to it."

DEFENSIVENESS. Remember when I said you can make people feel bad about what they're doing just by doing what you're doing? Picture this: You roll up to the lunch table at work and pull out your leftover peppers stuffed with ground chicken, sweet onions, roasted tomatoes, and cauliflower rice. And a small container of homemade pesto. And a bottle of kombucha. They're all eating cold pizza and drinking soda. It's like Molly Ringwald in *The Breakfast Club* showing up to detention with sushi in her lunch box. Then the comments come rolling in.

"Oh, don't look at my soda, it'll make your pancreas hurt."

"It must be nice to have all that time to cook."

"Want some pizza? Of course you don't!"

Your own healthy food choices and commitment to change acts as an unintentional mirror, reflecting their own poor choices back at them. And sometimes their ensuing frustration will be taken out on you. It's enough to make you want to eat alone at your desk . . . but you shouldn't. Try to remember: This isn't about you, it's about them and their discomfort with their own less-than-healthy habits. It's not like you're being judgmental, critical, or preachy about your new healthy diet and their less-than-stellar habits.

Wait, you're not, right?

MIRROR CHECK

Take a good, hard look at this one. Are you, perhaps, being a little judge-y or preachy with these folks, even if you mean well? Comments like "I bet you'd like sparkling water just as much as soda," or "I had no idea how gross pizza was making me feel until I stopped eating it" may be intended as helpful, but will only come across as passive-aggressive, especially if your dining-mates are already feeling a little uncomfortable with their choices. The best policy here is still not to talk about food over food, and never to offer anyone unsolicited advice on their dietary habits. Like, ever. Just don't.

Your strategy here is a one-two punch: deflect, then change the subject. Make it clear that their food choices aren't even on your radar, and there are much more interesting things to talk about than what's on everyone's plate. It sounds like this: "Ha! Don't you worry about my pancreas. How did your presentation go?" Or "Yeah, this is one of my favorite meals these days. Did your son win his soccer game?" Or "No, thanks, but I do want to hear all about your date last night."

It's quick. It's direct. You're not getting defensive or responding with something that could stoke the fire even more. (Like, don't say, "I *make* time to cook, Karen. I have the same twenty-four hours as you." Even if you want to. Be the bigger person here.) If they repeat their remarks, stick to your strategy, ignore or deflect, and change the subject. If it gets really bad or they start ganging up on you, excuse yourself for a minute to get some water, check a text, or use the bathroom. Buy yourself some space, let the conversation move on, and return with a pleasant remark.

FEELING LEFT BEHIND OR JEALOUS. This one is especially common with women and their girlfriends but can happen with any group or pairing where food plays a big part in your relationship. Maybe you always meet for drinks after work, or have an indulgent weekly brunch date, or a habit of breaking out the ice cream when discussing your dating troubles. Now that you're changing your diet, these people feel like they may be tossed out right along with the wine/French toast/Rocky Road—as if your friendship or relationship can't survive without a solid foundation of comfort food and treats.

They may also be plain old jealous of both your newfound motivation and the attention you may be getting as the result of your efforts. To the outside world, your dedication is impressive and your enthusiasm is contagious; even your lunches are envy-worthy these days. Not to mention that you're looking leaner, your skin is glowing, you've got more confidence, and you've started chatting up that cute I.T. tech at lunch.

What if people start paying all this attention to you? What if you decide you need new friends who are just as health-conscious as you? *What if you start doing triathlons?*

It's all terrifying, and your friends, family, or co-workers might not handle these fears well. The comments may sound a lot like defensiveness: "I wish I could afford to shop at the health food store" or "Yeah, it'd be easier if I still lived at home like you do." They may also try to bring you down to size or remind you that you haven't always been so healthy—low blows that could jeopardize your growth mind-set. It might sound like this:

"You've lost some weight, maybe . . ."

"You're not as fun when you're not drinking."

"Don't forget that just last month you pigged out on nachos, too."

"You're just not the same now that you're doing this new diet."

Ouch. Just remember, the peanut gallery comments aren't about you, they're about the peanut gallery and their own fears, insecurities, and unhappiness with their own habits.

They're coming from a highly emotional place, and all you can do is reassure them through your words and actions and maintain as "normal" a friendship as you can while they get used to your new dietary habits and healthy lifestyle. Move interactions with these people away from food and into other areas of shared interest. Don't meet for lunch; schedule a pedicure, a trip to the bookstore, a basketball game, or a hike instead. (Make sure it's actually a shared interest—suggesting you go to a yoga class when the other person doesn't know down-dog from a hot dog isn't going to help your cause.) This will help you avoid the highly charged environment of a restaurant or dining room table, and give you time and space to reinforce all the other ways you two can connect and have fun.

Then just keep on keepin' on, and in the meantime, continue to be the best friend, family member, or co-worker you can. Work extra-hard not to let your dietary changes get in the way of your friendship, because then your critics will be justified in resenting your new habits. "I'd love to go to dinner, but it's so hard to go out with this new diet" isn't going to win you any points, and it only reinforces the idea that you really are changing the course of your friendship. Accept invitations for drinks, and just matter-of-factly order water. Enjoy the birthday party, but pass on the cake. Have people over for dinner, cook them a delicious meal, and don't even mention this is how you're eating every day on this new "diet." Once they see that your relationship isn't going to change just because you're eating healthy foods, things should get back normal.

FEAR OF REJECTION. Remember when I said food isn't just food; it's also love, and sometimes the only way two people have been able to bond or come together? Now imagine that Mom's cookies, Gram's lasagna, and your co-worker's Friday morning "I brought bagels!" are no longer a conduit for connection because they're not part of your reset. Cue hurt feelings, withdrawal of affection, and lots of taking it personally.

You're just declining their offer of food, but it feels like you're rejecting *them.*

This is especially hard with mothers, because your history with your parents and food are long-standing, habits are well established, and patterns are subconscious. You don't think about the fact that your mom bakes for you when she's feeling neglected, or needs to have a hard conversation, or just wants to feel like she's still your mom even though you moved out years ago. It's what she's always done, and all of a sudden you're saying no to her emotion-frosted peanut butter cookies.

Chances are, the folks who will feel personally rejected when you change your diet have their own dysfunctional relationships with eating. They can't separate the foods they make you from the emotions or connections they foster, and they may be insecure enough in your relationship to feel like their food is necessary for you to love them back.

Your job here is to gently remind them otherwise.

First, if you haven't already, be specific about why you're passing on these foods during your reset. Make it as personal as is appropriate for your relationship. With moms, get *into* it. Show her that you can connect through authenticity and vulnerability, not just cookies. "Mom, I still love your cookies, but I've been totally out of control with my sugar consumption. Even when I tell myself 'not tonight,' I can't stop eating ice cream or chocolate. It makes me feel awful about myself, and it's really hurting my self-esteem. I'm doing this reset so I can get back in control and enjoy things like your cookies without going totally off the rails, but that means passing on them for now."

Explain your reasoning in a way that shows your common ground, like a shared frustration with allergies, energy levels, joint pain, or sleep quality. Tell her how your struggles are making you feel, opening up to her in a way that creates a shared bond. Remind her that your reset diet isn't forever—it's just a short-term experiment to help you figure out how these foods are affecting you. And if you're already experiencing benefits from your reset, share that, too! Let her know you're missing these foods, but the results so far are encouraging you to stick with it.

Then find other ways to connect: Play a game, go for a walk, schedule a spa day, attend a sporting event, go play outside, watch a movie—anything that you both enjoy that doesn't have to do with less-healthy food. If cooking and eating are significant areas of bonding for you, keep doing that—just suggest a different meal. "I'm passing on lasagna right now, but your chicken cacciatore has always been a favorite. Can you make that for me instead?" (Or better yet, offer to make it together.)

Finally, *do* stay connected. If their primary fear is rejection, disappearing for weeks at a time during your reset isn't going to help your situation. Make an effort here. Send photos of your hike, the last book you read, or a recipe that you'd both enjoy. E-mail status updates on how good you're feeling and the non-scale victories you're racking up. Schedule visits, make time for short chats, send cards in the mail—anything to reinforce the idea that your relationship isn't dependent on food.

Threat Level: Orange

Sometimes, all the patience, empathy, and consideration in the world won't derail your friends, family, or co-workers from being jerk-faces about your new healthy habits. I hope you never encounter this, but here's what you might experience:

- **They're constantly tempting you with things you "can't" eat or drink.**

- They purposefully try to make you feel bad for declining their offers of less-healthy fare.

- They go out of their way to make you feel different or weird for your eating habits.

- They always choose social locations that are not conducive to your health concerns, like pizza parlors or the local bar.

- When dining at their homes, they never prepare options that you can enjoy (or bother asking if there is anything special you need).

What the hell, Becky?

If this is what's happening, your first inclination may be to launch a full-scale defense, but that move is guaranteed to continue the conflict. Let's just start off small by first repeating the original tactic I outlined: evade and redirect. Let them know your food choices are not up for discussion at the table. Then immediately change the subject. You can make it light, like, "I'm just trying to keep the grilled chicken people in business. Did anyone see the game last night?" You can speak plainly: "I really don't like talking about food over food. Let's just enjoy the meal—has anyone seen the new Superman movie?" You can be really up front: "I get it, you don't understand my new diet, but now is not the time to talk about it. Dad, how's the lawn coming along?"

This should at least get you through the meal, after which you can field questions in a more relaxed environment using all the techniques I've outlined in this book. Unless people are really dense. Or really mad at you for being so grossly healthy. Or if they've been drinking, in which case, you may need to take it a step further and address their rude behavior. If that's what you're forced to do, be direct, and be impassive. Say your piece, and then let it rest. Resist the urge to hammer them with example after example. Do not point out their own dietary shortcomings or actually call them jerk-faces. Try these:

YOU: "Every time I come out to eat with you, you give me a hard time about what I order. That's not cool. I don't care what you eat, and I expect you not to criticize me, either."

"You may not want to do what I'm doing, but I told you I'm in this for the full thirty days. Stop trying to get me to break my commitment—that's not okay."

"You know I'm not drinking this month, and I don't appreciate the high school–style peer pressure. Give it a rest, because I'm here to socialize and have fun, just like you."

Calling them out (especially if it's in front of others in your group) may be enough to get them to acknowledge their behavior and stop . . . or it might not do anything at all. Either way, do your best to keep your cool here, because if you come back with, "You know why I'm not drinking, Tom? Because *it makes you LOUD AND ANNOYING*," chances are you two aren't going to be BFFs for much longer. Which may not be a bad thing, because Tom isn't being a very good friend anyway.

If all else fails, again, be prepared to fall back. Are they really a valued friend or colleague if they won't respect your wishes and are constantly trying to undermine your efforts? I don't care how committed and self-confident you're feeling now; day after day after day of pressure and criticism like this will eventually get to you, and could compromise all the progress you've made.

Don't let that happen.

You are responsible for your own success here, and sometimes that means cutting people out of your life who just want to weigh you down. Hopefully, it's only temporary, and they'll realize they weren't being very supportive and come back around with a better attitude. Just remember one thing:

It's not you.

You're not the weird one, you're not the un-fun one, you're not the one spoiling the party by passing on the sangria. You should never feel bad about taking steps to make yourself healthier, and you should never let anyone (friend or otherwise) tell you differently.

There's also nothing wrong with making some new like-minded friends. As your hobbies and interests change, it's only natural that your circle of friends will expand to accommodate your new lifestyle. Look for people who are supportive and encouraging of your efforts, enjoy the same healthy pursuits, and will reinforce your growth mind-set. You can find these future friends anywhere and everywhere: in the gym, at the beach, on a hike, at a sporting event, or dining at the table next to you. (Restaurants—especially packed ones with closely set tables or places with communal seating—are the perfect way to connect; if the plate of the person next to you looks like yours, strike up a conversation.) Get comfortable chatting up strangers—it's not as hard as it sounds. "Burger no bun, that's how I order mine, too. Is this your go-to place for burgers?" or "I'm always looking for new hikes, what are some of your favorites?" are great conversation-openers and may lead you to a new friend or, at the very least, some new, healthy resources in your community.

GO VIRTUAL

Remember, when reality bites, you can boost your support system virtually by connecting with people through online forums, Facebook groups, and social media feeds. While these Interweb friends can't replace the oxytocin-boosting, stress-modulating impact of real-life social interaction, the more people you have in your corner, the better—especially if your corner at home is feeling kind of empty these days.

How Not to Win Friends and Influence People

You've been following all these strategies for communicating your food freedom hopes to the people you love. You're speaking from the heart, inviting them to witness your transformation and share in the health and happiness you've found through the process. These are magical moments, not unlike those feminine protection commercials where two besties run hand in hand through a sunlit field of daisies. Or something.

Sometimes, though, you try *so hard* to share your authentic experience with others that you turn your reset into a big ol' bummer for everyone around you—and invite the very pushback you are trying to avoid. The worst part is, you don't even realize you're doing it; all you know is that you're feeling even more isolated and anxious around food. So before we close this chapter out, let's talk about the ways *you* may be the one messing this thing up, and how to maybe not do that, m'kay?

COMPLAIN CAREFULLY. In an effort to "be real" and share your authentic experience—the good stuff and the not-so-good stuff—you turn into a giant complainer, making everyone in your life hate the very idea of food freedom and prompting communal eye-rolling any time you get around food. During happy hour: "I miss wine so much." At family dinner: "That lasagna looks so good. I'll just eat my salad and be sad." At the birthday party: "I *really* want cake, but I have two more days on my reset, so I can't." Womp womp.

Yes, you're being authentic, but "authentic" doesn't mean "verbally vomit every thought inside your head RIGHT THIS MINUTE." You may think you're just keeping it real by letting them know that sometimes it's hard, but all you're doing is making your reset sound Debbie Downer miserable, and reinforcing their preconceived notions that this new "diet" is nothing but hanger and deprivation.

LESSON: Whine with caution. It's okay to grumble during difficult moments, but be judicious about where, when, and with whom you choose to share those thoughts. Find someone who is already supportive of your efforts, and let her know up front that you're just venting—the majority of the time, you love what your reset is bringing you. Type out your temper tantrums in an online forum or Facebook group full of people who have been there, done that, and will understand that sometimes, it sucks. Or journal your innermost negative thoughts, because getting it down on paper is often enough to make you feel better. Finally, yes to sharing authentically, but no to dropping your temporary frustrations on an unprepared party, especially if they're not around to see all the moments throughout the day when you're actually really happy with your chosen path. You don't want to give them the wrong idea of food freedom, especially if you hope they'll someday join you in the journey.

DON'T BE PREACHY. You love your reset. You love it SO MUCH. And you think everyone in the whole world should do it, because it will change their life, too. So you tell them. Everyone. Anyone. All the time. You turn into a one-man (or woman) food freedom fanatic, because in your enthusiasm you really think you're being oh so helpful.

It's probably totally coincidental that your co-workers are always rushing back to their desks as soon as you walk into the breakroom.

While your intentions are good, constantly suggesting that your loved ones would look and feel much better if they only did what you are doing only pushes them further away. Keep it up, and you'll eventually find yourself totally isolated, because people don't want to socialize with you if you're always criticizing their food choices, acting smug with your healthy plate, or giving them solutions to problems they're not ready to admit they have.

LESSON: You can't do it for them, and the only person you are responsible for in this process is you. Lead by quiet example. Let your reset results speak for themselves. Have compassion, because you know how hard it is to address your health, habits, and relationship with food. Let them come to you—and if they don't, that's none of your business anyway. This can be hard when the person you love is clearly struggling, but there are more effective ways of being supportive than shoving your belief system (and lettuce wraps) down their throats.

STOP APOLOGIZING. In an effort to be accommodating, you find yourself apologizing for your "weird diet" at every turn. You offer lengthy explanations for why you're not helping yourself to a bagel, ordering a glass of wine, or having dessert. You hold up the entire table by thanking the waiter profusely for accommodating your difficult order. Every time food appears, you tense up, waiting for everyone's eyes to move to your plate. You *really* don't want to be "that person."

Except no one cares what you're eating, or not eating. In fact, you're the only one making a big deal about it, and you're actually making things uncomfortable for everyone. Your behavior draws people's attention to you and your food, and instead of coming across as gracious, people will think you're not satisfied with your choices, and that taking on a reset makes socializing really difficult.

LESSON: Get comfortable with the idea that this is just how you're eating. The vegetarian doesn't apologize profusely for ordering a salad, the nonsmoker doesn't justify his refusal of a cigarette, and you don't need to say a thing when ordering sparkling water instead of wine. Thank your waiter for getting your "add this, none of that" order right (a generous tip works here) or your co-worker for remembering to order fruit along with bagels for your business meeting, but understand that you have nothing to apologize for. Show everyone that you can eat well and enjoy social occasions effortlessly, even if you have to fake the "effortless" part for a while. (Speaking of socializing ...)

GET OUT THERE. You are rocking your reset. Making good food choices feels effortless; you've settled into an easy routine of shopping, meal prep, and cooking; and you're racking up non-scale victories left and right. Everything is *so* good, in fact, that you don't want to tempt fate—so you find reasons to avoid happy hour, dinner parties, and brunch invitations. You eat at your desk rather than in the breakroom, where leftover pastries from the management meeting beckon. You'd love to visit your mom, but her house is full of temptation, so you put it off for another week. In fact, you put off all your socializing for just another week, or maybe two . . . just until you're feeling more secure in your food freedom.

Except now you've completely isolated yourself, demonstrating to friends and family that food freedom is actually a prison sentence, reinforcing the notion that doing a reset is incompatible with socializing, and making it clear that sticking to the plan is more important than your relationships.

LESSON: It's not exactly "freedom" if you place yourself in solitary confinement. Not only that—how are you supposed to learn how to stick to your reset in the real world if you're never out there *in* the real world? Tough love time: Don't be such a scaredy-cat. Food (or your friends and family) aren't out to get you, and you've got a dozen strategies for talking to others about the program. Don't deprive yourself of the fun—get out there and socialize! Bonus: In-person socialization is a powerful moderator of stress, which means the benefits you'll get from laughing, talking, and dining with those you love can help you relax into your reset that much more.

To Be Continued . . . in Life After

Congratulations! Your reset and reintroduction are over, and you've been successful in sharing your journey with those closest to you, recruiting their support and sharing all the benefits of your healthy-eating intervention.

Now comes the hard part.

Dealing with family and friends *during* your reset is actually pretty easy compared to life after. During your reset, you have a clear set of rules to follow, with little to no gray area. You've got the science of an elimination diet backing you up, and a reintroduction plan as reassurance that these food choices aren't set in stone forever. And if push comes to shove and you find yourself under serious pressure, just blame me. "Look, I committed to this, but that woman who wrote the book has eyes *everywhere*, so I am not going out to a glass of cheap wine."

I will neither confirm nor deny that I see all, but #WWMHD (*What Would Melissa Hartwig Do*) is an actual thing.

After your reset, however, you'll no longer have the rules, your 30-day commitment, or me to fall back on. This is the best part of your journey (enjoying your food freedom), but also the hardest to explain to others.

Happily, I can help you here, too.

CHAPTER 13

POST-RESET PREDICAMENTS

In other people's eyes, the day your reintroduction ends could be viewed as the dietary equivalent of school letting out for the summer. They may still be thinking about what you've been doing as a traditional "diet," despite your best efforts to explain how a reset is different. Even if they were supportive during the program, there's a good chance they're imagining you counting down the days until it's over, just like *they've* been counting down the days until they get their drinking/pizza/cookie-baking buddy back.

Here's what they're thinking: *You've waited this long. You must have been feeling so deprived. Surely you've missed these foods.* But they just offered you a beer/slice of pizza/half their cupcake, and you declined. Cue a tsunami of confusion.

THEM: But your diet is over.

YOU: Yeah, it's technically over.

THEM: But you still don't want this?

YOU: No, I actually don't.

THEM: But it's your favorite.

YOU: Yeah, it used to be.

THEM: So it's not anymore?

YOU: No, I guess it's not.

THEM: Who are you and WHAT HAVE YOU DONE WITH MY FRIEND?

This is the hard part—conveying to people that "reset" isn't just a noun, but a verb, too; you truly have *reset* your health, habits, and relationship with food, and you're actually *not* the same person as you were going into this. Your tastes are different, you feel like a million bucks, and you've made some connections between certain foods you used to eat and less-than-desirable effects on your body and brain. But these aren't changes people can see, and if they haven't been with you every step of the way, it can seem abrupt. They'll be disappointed, confused, and potentially annoyed.

It's like "What the hell, Becky," but *now you're Becky.*

However, as important as it is, this chapter is short, because you've already got the two previous chapters to help you explain your ongoing Food Freedom plan to friends, family, and co-workers.

First, borrow approaches from your reset conversations. Keep it positive. Focus on your personal experience. Be specific about the benefits of your reset, what you learned about how specific foods effect you, and (most critical) how you'll be using that information in Life After.

Here's how it might sound:

YOU: "My reset was such a great experience. I have more energy than I've had in years, my cravings are all but gone, and I lost six pounds without counting calories. During the process, I figured out that

cheese makes my skin break out and gluten really upsets my digestion. Now that I know this, I'm going to generally avoid these foods
unless it's something really incredible."

"I thought I'd miss alcohol during my reset, but I really didn't! I had
great energy, I slept so much better, and I made it to the gym way
more often. For now, I'm going to limit wine to special occasions,
because I just feel so much better when I'm not drinking."

"During my reset, I finally got my cravings under control and broke my
late-night snacking habit. I realized during reintroduction that eating
chocolate, chips and salsa, or anything sweet late at night makes me
want to stuff my face with sugar, so I'm going to be really careful about
treats going forward, especially after dinner."

CHOOSE YOUR WORDS CAREFULLY

Notice that in the examples, you're not saying, "I don't eat gluten now," "I'm not drinking alcohol anymore," or "No more
desserts for me." Unless you had such a terrible reaction to
a specific food during reintroduction that you'll be avoiding it at all
costs, don't use absolutes. It's far more likely that you'll still be eating
most foods occasionally, when they're worth it. Take some time now to
explain the concept of "worth it" and what that means to you. This will
help you avoid appearing hypocritical when you pass on the bread basket three times during dinner, then order chocolate cake for dessert.

Be clear that it's a process and that you're still not sure exactly how it's
going to look a month from now, never mind in six months. Let them know
you'll be creating and revising your plan as you go, so you reserve the right
to change your mind about whether something is "worth it." Share the three-
step Food Freedom program with them, letting them know that sliding back
into old habits is actually expected and part of the learning process. Explain
the tools you'll be using to prevent that, and that you've got realistic expectations about your new lifestyle. This reassures them that you're not just setting
yourself up for failure, as they've observed with every other diet you've tried.

A word of caution: There's a chance you'll come out of your reset feeling so strong, craving-free, and in control that you'll want to make grand proclamations like, "I don't even want that stuff anymore!" This will be met with a reasonable degree of skepticism. More likely, they'll just raise their donut in your general direction and laugh, "Talk to me in a week, bro." As excited as you are, temper your enthusiasm with a healthy dash of reality. Let them know that you don't expect to remain in perfect control from here on out and that a return to old behaviors and comfort foods will probably happen at some point, but you're fully prepared to handle it when it does. Emphasize that you're fully committed to following the plan, so slips no longer mean abandoning your healthy eating efforts and giving into the "What the Hell" effect.

That last part is critical. You want your loved ones to know that this time, your expectations are realistic, but that you're also in this for the long haul—that it's a lifestyle shift in the truest sense of the word. When people do see you slipping back into old habits, they don't have to worry that your "failure" will prompt an emotional month of binging and self-hatred. This will also keep them from thinking a slip means they *finally* have their drinking/pizza/cookie-baking buddy back, ramping up the peer pressure and making your return to the reset that much harder.

Then, especially if they're a major part of your support system or have expressed interest in trying the program, keep them apprised of what you're doing and how it's going. Sharing your journey as you flex your worth-it skills, start to slide back into old habits, and recover gracefully will not only help them better support you, but demonstrate continued commitment to and happiness with your new healthy lifestyle—and may finally inspire them enough to give it a shot for themselves.

Three Little Words

Despite the effectiveness of these conversations, you'll still need in-the-moment strategies for helping you stay true to your food freedom goals. Are you ready for a concept that could legitimately change your life, should you choose to embrace it? (Seriously. Wait for it.) Introducing the three most powerful words in your Food Freedom language:

No, thank you.

Three little words, which form a complete sentence in and of themselves, with no further requirement to explain, justify, or defend. Three gorgeous words, which, said simply and politely in response to a variety of situations, can take a potentially complicated or uncomfortable food situation and turn it into a total nonstarter.

"Would you like a glass of wine?"

"No, thank you."

"Have a slice of pizza."

"No, thank you."

"Can I cut you a piece of birthday cake?"

"No, thank you."

"Do you want some bread?"

"No, thank you."

The applications are endless, and crazy liberating. Because literally, THAT IS ALL YOU HAVE TO SAY. You may have to say it more than once, but that's okay. Just repeat after me: "No, thank you." And then smile. And then move on. If they ask why, you still don't have to defend your decision. You can simply say, "I just don't want one, thanks" or "Not tonight, but thanks." If your conversation partner is genuinely curious as to why you are declining but it's not a good time to get into it, you can say, "I'll explain later, but for now, no, thank you."

IT'S AMAZING.

Maybe they were trying to get a reaction out of you. Maybe they were genuinely confused about your refusal. Maybe they think you're just trying to be polite, but it's really okay if you have some. Regardless, in the face of multiple polite, smiling "No, thank yous," the other person will give up their crusade, and you'll be out of a potentially sticky situation gracefully.

I told you. CRAZY LIBERATING.

This idea might make you uncomfortable, like you're being rude. Or maybe you just feel the need to explain yourself in any situation. Or maybe you feel defensive because you're not quite used to your new habits yet, either. But adding on to your "No, thank you" can actually make the situation *worse*, not better. Observe:

YOU'RE UNCOMFORTABLE. Maybe a simple "No, thank you" makes you feel rude, so you decide to explain why you don't want the pizza/bread/wine. "No, thank you. I just did this thirty-day reset, and now I feel amazing and

I'm just thinking that if I eat pizza I'll probably get a stomachache, not that it's not good pizza, I'm sure it's really good, but pizza just doesn't agree with me, which I didn't know before, isn't that weird?" Yeah, that's *much* more comfortable.

LESSON: Remember, if you don't make a big deal out of it, other people will be less likely to as well. If your "no, thank you" really isn't enough, you can always add generic qualifiers: "I'm not that hungry right now" or "I'm just not feeling it tonight." But really, I encourage you to practice "No, thank you" as a stand-alone sentence.

YOU NEED AN EXCUSE. Some of you feel the need to justify your decisions. For everything. Always. So you may be tempted to make an excuse for your refusal of a particular food or drink. "Oh, I'd love a margarita, but I have to get up early tomorrow to practice my presentation, so I really can't." It seems like a nice, neat explanation will help your cause, but all you've really done is given your friend a problem to fix. "I'll come by tomorrow and help you practice—you'll get it done twice as fast. Now how about just one margarita?" Now you're in a tough spot, where you'll either have to make up *another* excuse, or accept a margarita you don't really want to drink because this is just getting awkward.

LESSON: Don't lie or pin your decision on anything other than what you want (or don't want) in this moment. Trust yourself, and let your decisions stand for themselves. Even if you do have a valid reason for declining, simply declining needs to be enough of a reason for family and friends to graciously accept your answer and move on.

YOU'RE ALREADY DEFENSIVE. This is common when you're new to the reset and food freedom. You're not totally entrenched in these new habits yet, and you feel like a bit of an imposter turning these things down now in the name of health and happiness when you used to eat them all the time. But if you come out of the gate charging—"No, thank you. You *know* I've been trying to eat healthier, and I *told* you that dairy makes me break out."—the entire situation will escalate, your conversation partner shooting back (a well-deserved), "Wow, okay SORRY" or "What crawled up your butt?"

LESSON: Get comfortable with your new, healthy habits, because this is just who you are now, and there is nothing to defend. Go back to the smoking scenario: If you used to smoke and then you quit, when people asked if you wanted a cigarette, you'd simply say, "No, thanks." The end. Now channel that, because you can do the exact same thing when declining fast food, junk food, candy, or alcohol.

Okay, now the exception to the rule: If a simple "no, thank you" is going to hurt someone's feelings, you owe it to them to qualify your response. This happens a lot with family, and I've faced this very situation myself. My mom came to visit earlier this year and brought a tin full of homemade "hermits": gingersnap-esque diagonally sliced* walnut-and-raisin-bedaz- zled treats from heaven. Or in this case, New Hampshire. Normally this would incite a barrage of text messages from me to my sister ("PROOF Mom likes me better") and several cookies happily savored with my morn- ing decaf. But this visit, I was in the middle of a work project and stressed from tons of travel. I couldn't afford to compromise my energy or health the way I know gluten + sugar would do, so I had to decline. She brought these all the way across the country just for me, and I said, "No thanks, Mom."

In this situation, a qualifier was in order.

Using all the skills I talked about in chapters 11 and 12, I explained to my mom the challenges I was facing, and how I know these amazing treats would negatively impact my focus and energy. I made sure she knew how much I loved her for thinking of me and how much I was bummed to miss out on them. I promised to save a few, because they'd still be good in a few days, and maybe by then this work project would be over and I could relax. And I shared them with my friends, who were more than thrilled to take them off my hands.

It turned out fine; Mom was cool about it, and it wasn't a big deal.

To Eat or Not to Eat?

But what if it actually *was* a big deal? There will be times when you will come to a food freedom crossroads. Option A: Eat something that you know will make you significantly less healthy and isn't worth it. Option B: Hurt someone's feelings in a major way. Both of these choices stink, but unless you're prepared to climb out the bathroom window in your party clothes, you're gonna have to choose one.

---

* Diagonally cutting a delicious treat makes it 34 percent more delicious, #science.

ALLERGY ALERT

Please don't drop the "A" word unless you actually do have a legitimate, diagnosed allergy. It might seem tempting to catch their attention with "I have an allergy" instead of saying you have a sensitivity or strong preference, but an actual allergy is serious business; serving someone a food to which they are allergic could literally kill them. Crying wolf with "allergies" too often will make restaurant servers, co-workers, and others who dine with you take the concept less seriously, which spells trouble for someone with an actual allergy or serious immune response (like celiac disease). It's better to be honest; "It's not an allergy, but I am sensitive, so I would prefer to avoid all cheese, milk, cream, or butter in my meal. Is there any dairy in this meal that I'm not seeing?"

First, if the food in question is going to seriously affect your health, as is the case with an allergy, intolerance, or known sensitivity, then you *must* speak up. Nobody wants you to be miserable for their sake, and they probably didn't realize (or forgot) that you don't tolerate this food well. Politely decline, and explain why without getting too graphic. "I wish I could, but I'm dairy-intolerant, so I'll have to pass," or "It looks delicious, but gluten gives me a migraine, so I'll decline." Be firm about this; you're talking about something that could have a serious impact on your health, and you must stick up for yourself.

If it's just a matter of preference, you'll have to make a judgment based on how badly it will mess you up versus how hurt or offended the serving party will be. Some factors to consider:

- **What are the actual consequences?** Being a little tired and bloated is different than knowing you'll spend the rest of the night in the bathroom or watch your joints swell before your very eyes if you indulge.

- **How special is the occasion?** A bar where a stranger buys you a glass of Chardonnay is totally different than your gram lovingly pulling your favorite, piping-hot apple pie out of the oven when you visit.

- **What kind of relationship do you have with this person?** I knew I could turn down my mom's hermits and she'd be okay with it, but if my new boss brought in a cake to celebrate my promotion, I'd think twice about refusing a slice.

If you choose to decline, feel free to offer an explanation like the one I gave to my mom. Keep it simple, thank them for the effort, and let them know why you won't be partaking. Use this as an opportunity to connect with the other person, sharing an important part of your life—your commitment to your health—with them. This is especially important if they cook for you often or you dine with them frequently. You don't want them making homemade pasta every time you come over, so be clear that this dish simply isn't something you can eat.

One simple statement you can pull out here with great effectiveness, even if you're talking to a total stranger: "It just doesn't work well for me." You don't have to go into detail; in fact, keeping it vague is often a sign that you'd rather *not* talk about the details and will encourage the other person to accept your response and move on. If they press you for more and you're not comfortable sharing the details, just turn it around and ask someone if they can find an example of this in their own lives. "Is there anything you don't eat, because it bothers you when you do? Maybe a particular vegetable or dairy product or something? Well, it's like that with me and bread."

On the other hand, sometimes you'll decide it's best to go with the flow, accepting the consequences in an effort to be a gracious guest or dining partner. You can accomplish this with minimum collateral damage, if you're smart about it. Accept a small serving; as little as you can get away with politely, or offer to share with someone. If it's dessert, this is easy—just cite being so full you only want a few bites. If it's wine or another alcoholic beverage, it's perfectly acceptable to say, "Just a splash, thanks." If it's a fixed portion served to you, eat enough so you're not totally wasteful and see if you can take the rest home, or ask a dining partner if they'd like to finish it for you.

Then just deal with the consequences—which will be nowhere near as serious as turning down the triple-layer chocolate cake your aunt Cathy spent the afternoon making just for you.

CHAPTER 14

IN CLOSING: GO BE FREE

While writing this book, I flew to New York City for some business meetings. It was technically winter but unseasonably warm; 65 degrees and sunny. It felt like the whole city was out and about, and since my meetings ended midday, I decided to partake in my favorite NYC activity: getting totally lost. I threw in my headphones, tied my Converse, and headed south with no particular destination in mind. I walked for two hours; past parks, stores, and restaurants, stopping anywhere that looked interesting.

And then, out of nowhere . . . CUPCAKE.

Allow me to transport you back to that day with me.

I'm heading back toward my hotel when I pass a little bakery with cupcakes in the window. I don't notice the name on the door, but it has pretty curtains, glows from the inside as if lit by angels, and I'm pretty sure I hear the cupcakes whispering my name.

It's not my birthday. It's not any sort of occasion. It's not even special that I'm in New York, because I'm there all the time. It's just 4 p.m. on a random Monday, the opportunity to eat a cupcake is upon me, and now I have to decide what to do.

Option 1: Go inside (which, let's be honest, translates to "Eat a cupcake").

Option 2: Heavy-breathe on the window until it gets awkward, then keep walking.

Here's how my Food Freedom plan goes down.

First, I know exactly how the sugar and gluten in the cupcakes will impact me, thanks to several resets and careful reintroductions. Calling on all my cupcake-eating experience (because reintroduction is a lifelong process), I'm able to predict that a cupcake means fighting with my Sugar Dragon for a few hours and being a little bloated for the rest of the night.

I also know that, for me, even one bite more than one cupcake tips the scale from "worth it" to "not worth it": a hard-earned lesson that finally solidified over New Year's 2014 when I threw down four cupcakes within a 24-hour period (including two for breakfast), without deliberation, consciousness, or control.

That was not as fun as it sounds.

Armed with that knowledge and thanks to all the "worth it" practice I'd done over the last seven years, I run through my food freedom checklist in a moment's time. I don't need to slow my breathing, give the cupcake a time-out, or walk around the block; after so much repetition, this evaluation happens automatically.

Is this cupcake truly special or delicious? I think it will be, yes.

Will it mess me up? Nothing I can't easily manage.

Is it worth it? Yes.

Do I really want it? Yes.

I also know from the mistakes I've made in the past (eating stuff that I told myself would be worth it, but wasn't), that if I had waffled on any of those answers, it's time to walk away. Those "mistakes" were actually valuable learning experiences, because now I know that if it's not a home-run on the first consideration but I eat it anyway, I'll end up regretting it.

So I go inside. It smells like vanilla and hugs.

Thinking back to my last birthday experience, I'm still asking myself, "Do I really want one?" as I look over all the flavors. It's still coming back "Hell, yes," so I carefully make my selection: vanilla, with chocolate buttercream frosting.

And sprinkles, because YOLO.

I leave the bakery with one cupcake, not two. (Suck it, Sugar Dragon.) I walk back to my hotel, trying not to squish the frosting. I have dinner plans soon, but I want the cupcake now.

I'm a grown-up. I can eat dessert first.

So I sit down in my hotel room with my cupcake. And by "sit down" I mean "climb into bed," because eating a cupcake in a fluffy hotel bed is about the most decadent thing I could imagine.

I open the box with reverence, lift out the cupcake, and take a bite.

The angels sing.

I take a photo of the cupcake and text it to a friend with the caption, "This. Is. Happening." That buys me some space and time to evaluate whether I need to eat more. I always follow the One-Bite Rule, still. I definitely want to eat more.

I take another bite. OMG, so good.

I eat the whole cupcake. I savor every bite. I save a huge gob of frosting and a tiny bit of cake for last. I take my time.

And then I stay in bed for a little while reading before I head off to dinner, where I order a Whole30-worthy meal, one glass of wine (worth it), and pass on the dessert menu, because nothing was going to be as good as that cupcake.

That is my food freedom.

Your Food Freedom

This book may be coming to a close, but your food freedom journey is just beginning. Here's what you have ahead of you. (Spoiler: It's awesome.)

You finish your reset looking and feeling better than you have in years, decades, maybe even ever. After successfully completing something that challenging, your self-confidence is through the roof. Your cravings are under control, and you're secure in your belief that you are a healthy person with healthy habits. You practically vibrate with energy. You look amazing. Everyone asks, "What have you been doing?"

You have a good idea of how the foods you've reintroduced will impact you. This makes it easier to avoid things that aren't going to be worth it, because a treat isn't really a treat if it's going to mess you up.

"WILL THIS MESS ME UP?"

Need a reminder of symptoms to look for here? Ask yourself these questions:

- Will it promote cravings or make my Sugar Dragon roar?

- Will it make me feel lethargic or put me on an energy roller coaster?

- Will it disrupt my sleep?

- Will it mess up my digestion or leave me with gas or bloating?

- Will it negatively impact my mood, attention span, focus, or motivation?

- Will it make my symptoms (pain, swelling, fatigue) flare up?

- Will it trigger an adverse reaction (asthma, migraines, skin breakouts)?

Thanks to the reintroduction process, you also bring some of the things you were missing on your reset back into regular rotation now that you know they don't negatively affect you. You happily start eating them again, without guilt or anxiety.

This is your food freedom: the perfect balance of healthy and less-healthy-but-worth-it foods, eaten in a way that is totally sustainable and keeps you feeling amazing.

When you come across something special or delicious, you use your food freedom tools to help you decide "yes" or "no, thank you," evaluating whether you really want it. You don't stress out about it, you simply think critically, comparing the potential benefits ("Is this going to taste as good as I imagine?") against the consequences ("Is this going to mess me up, physically or psychologically?"), and decide.

Worth it, or not worth it?

If it's not worth it, you simply pass. You don't feel deprived, because the decision was yours. If others question your choice, you use the conversation strategies you've learned to gain their support, or at the very least, honor your commitment to your goals. You walk away that much more secure in your food freedom.

This is winning.

If it *is* worth it, you accept. You savor. You enjoy it so hard. You eat as much as you need to satisfy the experience. Maybe that's a tiny sliver of office party birthday cake. Maybe it's of the entirety of That Cupcake In The Window. Maybe it's the gelato *and* the wine *and* the pasta *and* the bread on vacation in Italy. There are no hard-and-fast rules here, because you are always evaluating what you need to satisfy *that* experience in *that* moment, and as long as your decisions are conscious and deliberate, there are no wrong answers. (Just potentially unpleasant consequences—but you're prepared to deal with those.)

Whatever you decide, no matter how much you eat, you remain in control, because you're paying attention the entire time. Your second bite only comes after you decide you really want more; your seventh bite is just as savored as the first. When you've had enough, you lick your fingers, sigh contentedly, and go right back to your regularly scheduled dietary choices. You successfully deal with any consequences of your choice. You don't beat yourself up. There is no guilt.

This is also winning.

You feel like you could do this forever. In practice, you'll just do it for a while. At some point, something will send you back toward the Land of Old Habits. You find you don't feel as awesome and you're no longer totally in control.

But.

You don't panic. You don't feel like a failure. You don't wallow in your ice cream. You just return to your reset, already feeling better having taken the first step back towards food freedom.

You stay on your reset as long as you need to, but no longer; maybe that's 10 days, maybe it's 40. You successfully complete a full reintroduction, again. You're incredibly proud of yourself, again. Your self-confidence, energy, and waistline return. As with every reset, you learn even more about how food impacts you and apply that new knowledge to "life after," so your everyday food freedom diet works even better for you.

You spend more and more time enjoying your food freedom. The process will feel easier and easier. Weeks will pass, and you won't even think about it, because you're just living it. You don't need to belly-breathe or distract yourself, and you don't need to run past your checklist line-by-line; you just ask yourself, "Worth it?" and answer, "Yes" or "No, thank you."

More times than not, you get it right. When you don't, and it's not actually worth it, you just make note for next time, and move on.

No guilt. No failure. Just a learning experience.

In the months and years that follow, you return to your reset less often, and for shorter periods of time. Your definition of "worth it" evolves based on your experience, your goals, your life. You have fun with your food, seeing how far you can expand your food horizons and not stressing when you get it wrong. You are happy and healthy, enjoying your food but no longer controlled by it.

This is what your life could look like. This is what food freedom can bring you. You want this, and I really want you to have it.

Food Freedom Forever

You've got all the tools you need to create your own version of food freedom. You've learned strategies for staying in control while savoring all the foods you decide are worth it, both in the moment and big-picture. You know your triggers and have plans in place to return you to the food freedom path if you find yourself off track. You're sharing your healthy eating efforts with the people you care about in a way that brings you closer together and might even motivate them to embark upon their own food freedom journey.

All that's left is to give yourself a high five and keep working the plan.

Notice I didn't say "*follow* the plan" or "*stick to* the plan." To quote musical superstar Rihanna:

Work, work, work, work, work.

Which is the only part of that song I understand; thank goodness it's applicable.

It will be work. You will have to *actively* participate in every part of this process. You can't just show up at the gym and expect to get fitter—you need to actually flex your muscles. Same here. Reading this book is a great first step. Completing a reset is huge. But that's only the very first part of this journey. Now you must work.

Pay attention. Think before you eat. Reflect on your choices. Journal. Commit to the process every single day. Even on vacation. Even when you're stressed. Even when you're so over the idea of "awareness" and "worth it" that you think, "Screw it, I'm going to take the weekend off and come back to it on Monday."

Especially then.

It will get easier. You will move through the steps and strategies with more fluidity. When you veer off course, you will quickly find your way back. You will experience glorious moments where it's completely effortless; you automatically run through the process, make your choice, enjoy the hell out of it, and move on. This will feel amazing. Stop here, and let it feel amazing. You've earned that.

You will drink a glass of wine on your birthday, or two, or none, and you will be happy.

This can be your food freedom future, if you do the work.

This work will be significantly easier if you stay connected to the healthy-eating communities you joined during your reset. This is something you may not have even considered. The camaraderie of your online group during your reset was really helpful, but you've graduated now. It's a reset-focused support group, and you're done with your reset, so it's time to move on, right?

Oh so wrong.

Consider this tip your secret food freedom weapon: Post-reset, continue to comment on your favorite healthy-eating social media feeds, check in with people on the forum, and answer questions in your Facebook group. Share resources. Help new people. Talk about what "life after" looks like for you. Ask for help when you need it. These simple acts will provide a number of food freedom benefits.

FIND THE RIGHT SUPPORT

I f you find, post-reset, that you're no longer getting the right kind of support in your support group, don't be afraid to find another! Every forum, message board, and blog has its own dynamics and culture; finding the group that's right for you long term is critical. You may want to "audit" a few new communities before committing to any one group, or use different sites or feeds for different reasons: one to hold you accountable to your Food Freedom plan, one when you just need someone to tell you "good job," and another for when you're back on your reset protocol. Take as much time as you need here to find the right post-reset communities for you, because getting this right can make a huge impact on your continued food freedom success.

Staying connected with your reset support group reinforces your growth mind-set, reminding you that you're still a healthy eater with good habits, even though you occasionally eat (totally worth it) less-healthy foods. If you've connected with the right people, their offerings will make it easier to maintain your healthy habits, providing a wealth of delicious recipes, meal planning strategies, and cooking tips.

Offering advice to others through their reset might also make you feel really good. In fact, it could actually help you just as much as it helps them. Earlier this year, I jumped on the Whole30 Instagram account to provide guidance to a woman caring for a sick family member and beating herself up for her boring-but-still-compliant reset food choices. I advised her to shift her mind-set away from trying to do the "perfect" reset with fancy recipes and homemade everything; focusing instead on sticking to the rules 100% and being proud of herself for it—even if that involved a microwave, a grass-fed hot dog, and a paper plate.

As I typed this response, something clicked for me, too—this concept of letting good enough be good enough during times of stress, and the ways in which I could apply this in my own life while writing this book. This was when, as I mentioned earlier, I immediately stopped putting pressure on myself to cook (and Instagram) complicated recipes and started making variations of simple meals I could put together quickly but still really enjoy. My point is, you may also find yourself offering advice to someone else, only to realize that was *exactly* what you needed to hear, too—a major win-win for your food freedom.

Remaining involved in your community will also help prevent the dreaded slow slide (back on page 129), keeping you focused on and committed to working the program and accountable to your community for your choices.

It's hard to pretend all those grabbed-a-muffin-for-breakfast mornings aren't happening when people still want to know what you're eating and how it's going.

You can also reinforce your new relationship with food by expanding your focus and commitment to include other healthy pursuits, like exercise, sleep, or meditation. This often feels natural and intuitive; taking back control over food is a powerful experience, and the sense of self-confidence it brings will spill over into every other area of your life.

You'll watch less television. You'll take the stairs. You'll join a book club. You'll plant some herbs. You'll write in your journal. You'll try a yoga class. You'll meditate. You'll call your mother.

Bonus: Surrounding your food freedom with other healthy habits makes it easier to maintain them all. When you feel great, you'll be motivated not just to continue paying attention and working the plan, but to adopt other feel-good habits, like walking more, joining a gym, or taking that cooking class you've been wanting to try. Once you do those things, you will feel even healthier, and the lovely cycle will continue.

This is who you are now.

This is what you do now.

You are a healthy person, with healthy habits, living in true food freedom.

It makes me want to heart emoji.

I am so honored to be on this journey with you, and I wish you nothing but health, happiness, food freedom forever, and the occasional cupcake with two inches of frosting.

But only if it's worth it.

RESOURCES

Finding a Functional Medicine Practitioner

If you have a chronic health condition, are being treated for or take medication for a specific disease, or simply want to implement a reset plan specific to your unique health history and goals, I highly recommend seeking the help of a qualified functional medicine practitioner.

Functional medicine addresses the underlying causes of disease, using a systems-oriented approach and engaging both patient and practitioner in a therapeutic partnership. It is an evolution in the practice of medicine that better addresses the health-care needs of the twenty-first century. By shifting the traditional disease-centered focus of medical practice to a more patient-centered approach, functional medicine addresses the whole person, not just an isolated set of symptoms.

Functional medicine practitioners spend time with their patients, listening to their histories and looking at the interactions among genetic, environmental, and lifestyle factors that can influence long-term health and complex, chronic disease. In this way, functional medicine supports the unique expression of health and vitality for each individual.

Here are four websites designed to help you find a practitioner in your local community, and provide you with helpful tips for choosing and working with your new health-care provider.

INSTITUTE FOR FUNCTIONAL MEDICINE:
w30.co/whole30ifm

AMERICAN BOARD OF INTEGRATIVE HOLISTIC MEDICINE:
abihm.org/search-doctors

INTEGRATIVE MEDICINE FOR MENTAL HEALTH:
integrativemedicineformentalhealth.com/registry.php

PRIMAL DOCS:
primaldocs.com/members

Reset Diets

Here are several pre-designed reset options, and resources (websites, books, and more) for each.

Whole30

whole30.com

Created in 2009, the Whole30 is my 30-day program designed to push the reset button with your health, habits, and relationship with food.

This is the official home of the Whole30 program, where you'll find the free Whole30 Forum, PDF downloads, Whole30-Approved products and affiliates, and more Whole30-related articles than you could possibly hope to read in 30 days. Spend lots of time exploring here before, during, and after your Whole30—this is the very heart of our community.

Facebook: whole30

Instagram: @whole30, @whole30recipes, @whole30approved

Twitter: @whole30

Snapchat: whole30

YouTube: whole30

Pinterest: whole30

Books

The Whole30: The 30-Day Guide to Total Health and Food Freedom, by Melissa Hartwig and Dallas Hartwig

The Whole30 Cookbook, by Melissa Hartwig (December 2016)

It Starts With Food: Discover the Whole30 and Change Your Life in Unexpected Ways, by Dallas Hartwig and Melissa Hartwig

Paleo Autoimmune Protocol (AIP)

The Paleo AIP is a reset protocol designed specifically for those with autoimmune conditions like lupus, rheumatoid arthritis, PCOS, or Hashimoto's thyroiditis.

DR. AMY MYERS
amymyersmd.com
*The Autoimmune Solution: Prevent and Reverse the Full Spectrum
of Inflammatory Symptoms and Diseases*

SARAH BALLANTYNE, PHD
The Paleo Mom
thepaleomom.com
The Paleo Approach
The Paleo Approach Cookbook
The Healing Kitchen

MICKEY TRESCOTT
Autoimmune Paleo
autoimmune-paleo.com
The Autoimmune Paleo Cookbook
The Autoimmune Wellness Handbook (November 2016)

JESSICA FLANIGAN, CLINICAL NUTRITIONIST
AIP Lifestyle
aiplifestyle.com
The Loving Diet: Going Beyond Paleo into the Heart of What Ails You

Specific Carbohydrate Diet (SCD)

The Specific Carbohydrate Diet™ has helped many thousands of people with various forms of bowel disease and other ailments vastly improve their quality of life. It is a diet intended mainly for Crohn's disease, ulcerative colitis, celiac disease, diverticulitis, cystic fibrosis, and chronic diarrhea.

ELAINE GOTTSCHALL
Breaking the Vicious Cycle
breakingtheviciouscycle.info/home
Breaking the Vicious Cycle; Intestinal Health through Diet

JORDAN REASONER AND STEVE WRIGHT
SCD Lifestyle
scdlifestyle.com

GAPS Diet

The GAPS diet was derived from the *Specific Carbohydrate Diet* (SCD) to naturally treat chronic neurological conditions and inflammatory conditions in the digestive tract and as a result of a damaged gut lining and an imbalanced bacterial ecosystem within the GI tract.

DR. NATASHA CAMPBELL-MCBRIDE
gapsdiet.com
Gut and Psychology Syndrome

Low-FODMAP Diet

FODMAPs (Fermentable Oligosaccharides, Disaccharides, Monosaccharides, and Polyols) are a collection of fermentable carbohydrates and sugar alcohols found in foods. FODMAPs are poorly absorbed, thereby "feeding" gut bacteria and causing a host of symptoms, including gas, bloating, digestive distress, and systemic inflammation in sensitive individuals. A low-FODMAP diet may help reduce symptoms, and is often used to treat irritable bowel syndrome (IBS) or inflammatory bowel disease (IBD).

SUE SHEPHERD, PHD
Shepherd Works
shepherdworks.com.au
The Complete Low-FODMAP Diet: A Revolutionary Plan for Managing IBS and Other Digestive Disorders, with Peter Gibson, MD
The Low-FODMAP Diet Cookbook

PETER GIBSON, MD
Monash University
med.monash.edu/cecs/gastro/fodmap/
The Monash University Low FODMAP Diet Booklet

DR. BARBARA BOLEN
drbarbarabolen.com
The Everything Guide to the Low-FODMAP Diet

STANFORD UNIVERSITY MEDICAL CENTER
w30.co/stanfordfodmap
(comprehensive list of high- and low-FODMAP foods)

Connect with Melissa Hartwig

I'd love to see what you're eating on your reset, read your food freedom success stories, and hear what food freedom means to you. (Plus, I'm always good for some tough love if you need it.)

Instagram: @melissa_hartwig

Facebook: hartwig.melissa

Twitter: @melissahartwig_

Snapchat: @hartwig_melissa

Books on Habit and Change

Better Than Before, by Gretchen Rubin

The Power of Habit, by Charles Duhigg

The End of Overeating, by Dr. David Kessler

Switch, by Chip Heath and Dan Heath

You Are Not So Smart, by David McRaney

What Makes Your Brain Happy and Why You Should Do the Opposite, by David DiSalvo

The Willpower Instinct, by Kelly McGonigal

10% Happier, by Dan Harris

Loving What Is, by Byron Katie

INDEX

F

Facebook, 113
family. *See also* holidays; social
    connections
    fear of rejection, 206–7
    Food Freedom, talking about,
        138–39
    holiday meals, 138–40
    reset, talking about, 177–95
    resetting with, 165, 166
fat adaption, 48, 49
fats, high-fat diets, 51
feeling stuck, 157–59
Fermentable Oligosaccharides,
    Disaccharides,
    Monosaccharides, and
    Polyols (FODMAPs), 33, 35,
    50, 238
fitness trackers, 132
fixed mind-set, 104–5
Flanigan, Jessica, 237
flight attendants, cravings in, 60
FODMAPs (Fermentable
    Oligosaccharides,
    Disaccharides,
    Monosaccharides, and
    Polyols), 33, 35, 50, 238
food dyes, 33
food freedom, 77–85
    as conscious and deliberate, xvi,
        xvii, 79, 82–84
    enjoying food freedom, 78–80
    feeling in control, xix, 3
    food freedom cycle, 8
    as hard (but it gets easier), 7–8
    introduction, 3–9
    less bad isn't always good, 84
    as lifelong journey, 6–9, 72–73,
        81–82
    pay attention, 79–80
    questions to ask before
        consuming less-healthy
        options, 85

    social graces, 83
    3-step plan, 4–6
    "worth it" foods, 80–81
    your new way of eating, 7
food journals
    identifying slow slide, 130–31
    reintroduction process, 68–69
    reset process, 54
    sample, 131
food labels, 38, 42
friends. *See* social connections
fruit, dried, 42
functional medical practitioners, 32,
    72, 235

G

GAPS (Gut and Psychology
    Syndrome) Diet, 35, 238
Gibson, Peter, 238
girlfriends. *See* significant others
gluten
    Basic Reset, 52
    elimination diet, 33, 41
    physiological impact, 81
    pushback, 200
    reading labels, 42
    reintroduction, 64, 65, 67
    Vegan Reset, 50
goals
    diet goals, 18–19
    reset goals, 31, 41
Gottschall, Elaine, 237
grains
    Anti-Inflammatory Reset, 44
    Basic Reset, 52
    Craving-Buster Reset, 42, 43
    elimination diets, 33
    Energy Reset, 47, 48
    physiological impact, 34
    pseudo-cereals, 51
    reintroduction, 64, 65, 66, 67

and Sugar Dragon, 43
Vegan Reset, 50
Whole30 reset, 28
growth mind-set, 12, 104–6, 117
guilt and shame, 61, 94–96, 178
Gut and Psychology Syndrome
(GAPS) Diet, 35, 238
gut problems, 48, 50

H

habits. *See also* routines
overwriting old habits, 127–28
support from others, 56
time needed to make or break, 36
HAPIfork, 94
Harris, Dan, 117
Hartwig, Dallas, 12–13, 236
Hartwig, Melissa
books by, 236
drug addiction and recovery, 12
her story, 11–15
social media handles, 239
Whole30 development, 12–13
health-care practitioners
functional medical practitioners,
32, 72, 235
getting on board, 201
medical conditions and reset,
32, 39
"healthy person" mind-set, 95,
105–6, 108, 150, 228, 233
high-fat diets, 51
holidays. *See also* family
don't share specifics, 138
four-part game plan, 138–39
"if/then" plans, 140
indulging, 140–42
as trigger, 136–42
"worth it" foods, xvi–xvii, 83

home alone
binging, 150
"if/then" plans, 150
if you don't have it, you can't eat
it, 149
laziness, 148–49
as trigger, 147–51
husbands. *See* significant others

I

IBD (inflammatory bowel disease),
238
IBS (Irritable Bowel Syndrome),
diets for, 35, 238
"if/then" plans, 111–12, 140, 150
imagination, as success strategy,
89–90
immune system
Anti-Inflammatory Reset, 44–47
chronic inflammatory conditions,
35, 45, 238
stress response, 119
in-the-moment success strategies.
See success strategies, in-
the-moment
indulging. *See also* "worth it" foods
choosing not to, 140, 141
food journal, 131
on holidays, 140–42
one-bite rule, 91–92
regret, 96–98
return to regularly scheduled
diet, 98–99
savoring food, 90–91
success strategy, 90–94
inflammation, 35, 44–47, 238
inflammatory bowel disease (IBD),
238
iPhones. *See* smartphones
Irritable Bowel Syndrome (IBS),
diets for, 35, 238

J–K

L

M

N–O

P

concern for you, 202–3
countering arguments, 199–201
defensiveness, 203–4
don't apologize, 212
don't be preachy, 211
evade and redirect, 208
expect the best, 198
fear of rejection, 206–7
feeling left behind, 205–6
get out there, 212–13
go virtual, 210
jealousy, 205–6
mirror check, 204
peer pressure, 202–7
quoting science, 201
threat level: orange, 207–9
what not to do, 210–13

R

Readinger, Luc, 201
Reasoner, Jordan, 237
recipes, 47
regret, as inevitable, 96–98
reintroduction
    after mini reset, 162
    amounts, 81
    building a life of food freedom, 72–73
    changes to watch for, 66, 68
    vs. dieting, 60
    evaluating your reset, 70–73
    guidelines, 63–69
    guilt, 61
    ideas, 65
    journal, 68–69
    less healthy foods, 79–80
    as lifelong practice, 81–82, 97
    not missing it?, 68
    one food at a time, 62–63
    post-vacation, 136
    reinforcement, 62–63

sample schedule, 66–67
time required, 62
Whole30, 71
"worth it" foods, 79–81
relationships. See family; significant others; social connections
relationships with food
    difficulty of changing, 163–64
    and failure of diets, 20
    language of food, 94–96
    love-hate connection, 13
    yo-yo eating, 13–14
reset, initial, 23–57
    added sugar, 38
    Anti-Inflammatory Reset, 44–47
    Basic Reset, 52–53
    benefits, 54
    black-and-white rules, 39, 40
    carb-phobia, 49
    chronic systemic inflammation, 45
    common criticisms, 198–201
    Craving-Buster Reset, 8, 42–44
    cravings, 60
    dairy, 43
    decision factors, 24–25
    design your own, 31–33
    vs. diets, 21, 60
    duration, 35–36, 72
    elimination, 33–40
    Energy Reset, 47–49
    evaluation, 70–72
    in Food Freedom plan, 4–6
    foods to eat, 36–37
    goals, 31, 41
    medical conditions, 25, 32
    nightshades, 46
    non-scale victories, 33
    not quite vegan, 51
    often-problematic foods, 33–34
    planning your elimination, 35–39
    pre-big event, 144
    read labels, 38, 42

W

waiting period, as success strategy, 89

weighing yourself, 29, 32

"What the Hell" Effect
  and alcohol, 135
  birthdays, 141
  definition, 98
  holiday meals, 139
  post-reset predicaments, 218
  post-vacation, 135
  and stress, 142

whole grains. *See* grains

Whole30 program
  as anti-inflammatory diet, 44–45
  black-and-white rules, 40
  description and resources, 236
  "everything in moderation," 27
  overview, xix–xx, 26
  ready to try it?, 31
  as reset option, 5, 25–31, 71
  reset rules, 28–29
  specifics, 29
  support network, 27, 56
  testimonials, xix, 27
  as Vegan Reset alternative, 51
  you, on Whole30 reset, 30

willpower
  Basic Reset, 52
  boosting, 108–17
  daytime, 112
  diets, 17–18, 20

distraction techniques, 89
  and exercise, 115
  as finite, 20, 110
  "if/then" plan, 111–12
  and meditation, 116–17
  night before, 110–11
  and poor diets, 110
  positive thinking, 115
  and sleep, 111
  and stress, 120
  and technology, 112–14

wives. *See* significant others

The Work, 115, 121

workplace issues. *See* co-workers

"worth it" foods
  birthday indulgences, 140, 141
  changing definition of, 172–73
  communicating to others, 217
  definition, 80–81
  evaluation, 82, 85, 90, 100, 226–27, 228
  food freedom, 228–29
  less bad options, 84
  reevaluation, 92–93
  social situations, 83

Wright, Steve, 237

Y–Z

yo-yo resets, 166–67

Zen Habits website, 117